149 Ways
To Wipe Your Ass

(Observations of a Dermatologist)

Steven F. Wolfe, MD

Huzon Fyrst Press
Mooresville, NC

Author's Note

This book is a work of creative nonfiction. Some of the names of people and organizations in this story have been changed along with identifying details in order to protect their privacy. While I've tried to portray the events as accurately as possible, at times I condensed conversations or summarized scenes. Any inconsistencies or errors in this story are mine alone, though I'd like to blame them on I/T!

ISBN-13: 978-0-9970483-0-8

Produced in the United States of America

Huzon Fyrst Press
Mooresville, NC
149waystowipe@gmail.com

For Louie and Molly,
our beloved Keeshonds
who gave a decade and a half of love and licks

Contents

Part I

Ways to Wipe, Butts, Ass Kicking, Weiners
And Other Ways I See The World

Part II

How S&M, A Free Ticket to California,
And My 30 Days Of Addiction
Led Me To Become A Dermatologist

Part III

*Scrotal Surgery, Sterility, Paying For Sex
And More Observations*

Introduction

This book is about thinking. Thinking about what is important to you and what is not. What matters and what doesn't. It's about saying what's on your mind. It's about not being afraid to be critical. And it's about ripping apart things that annoy you, because that sometimes just makes you feel better or keeps you from going insane, especially when it has anything to do with I/T!

It's also about telling a story about situations that have mattered in your life. I hope that I stimulate you to think and that I touch your life by sharing what I wrote. And I hope that I haven't wasted your money buying this book.

One of my goals was to provide you, the reader, a value. Getting more out of reading and paying for this book than what you put into it (your time and money). At the very least, this book can be read in the bathroom! And if you don't like it, then take it on your next trip into the wilderness and it will become the 150th way to wipe your ass!

Part I

*Ways to Wipe, Butts, Ass Kicking, Weiners
And Other Ways I See The World*

Chapter 1

149 Ways
To Wipe Your Ass

S aturday mornings are a time when I typically have some downtime and the capacity to reflect on life in a bigger way than during the week. On a recent Saturday morning, I pondered the reasons why life really was better when I was growing up in the 1970s and 1980s.

There was no email, voicemail, internet or texting.

When you went on vacation, nobody could reach you—perfect, just what you wanted when you were on vacation—to forget about your daily grind. And when you returned from vacation, you didn't have 500 emails to go through because there were NO emails. Anywhere. Anytime.

There was no computer, laptop, tablet, iPhone 6, 5, 4, 3, 2, or 1. BLASTOFF.

If you wanted to know something, you went to the library, or your grandmother bought you an encyclopedia, or you asked someone, or it just didn't matter that you couldn't know everything on command. Or you did the obvious thing when someone asked you something, you made up the answer and they accepted it.

If you needed to get somewhere, you got in the car and *asked* when you got lost and then asked *again,* and you actually made it to your destination. Or you went to AAA and got a TripTik, and the other person in the car told you when and where to turn.

So why is your life so much worse today? Because your vacation is your work. You connect back every day. If you perhaps are a sanitation truck driver (no offense intended) and there is no need to connect back to *work*, you have other things to take up your time. You take a picture of your hotel room and post it to your Facebook account so 100 other people who have nothing better to do can look at your hotel room.

And every day you have to clear out clutter. Cut through the garbage. The 98% of things that don't matter so you can figure out the 2% of stuff that does matter like you forgot to pay your mortgage before you went on vacation. Or you actually just want to know the next lie that the government told so you are on www.msn.com or www.usatoday.com wasting more of your precious vacation.

Now you have to know everything every second and communicate it with someone else because you think someone actually cares. While driving, you have to post to Facebook that you love the song 'Happy,' then cross the median and hit a truck causing your car to catch on fire and kill you. (True Story--Highpoint, NC April 27, 2014).

Why is life so complicated? Here's why: Because when you go to the supermarket, you don't just have to decide on the brand of cereal you want, you have to decide the *type* of the brand. One common brand that used to just have the namesake of the brand, now has at least 16, yes 16 flavors. It comes in plain, honey nut, honey nut medley crunch, multigrain, multigrain peanut butter, multigrain dark chocolate crunch, apple cinnamon, cinnamon burst, protein cinnamon almond, protein oats and honey, ancient grains, chocolate, frosted, fruity, banana nut, and dulce de leche. This doesn't even include the discontinued burst varieties which included yogurt burst and 4 types of berry burst, namely strawberry, strawberry banana, cherry vanilla, and triple berry. The discontinued burst flavors alone are enough to burst my brain! Screw this. I don't even like cereal. Now I feel nauseous, and that taco I ate for dinner last night is running through me. I better go get some toilet paper.

I think I'll get my favorite brand. It's the one we got in the 1970s. The 4-pack. Hold on just a minute buddy. What's this? The *whole* aisle is now that brand's toilet paper? The other brands of toilet paper have their own aisles too? Well, here's my brand on aisle *number two*.

Let's see.......and gosh that taco is really moving now. Do I want the ultra strong, ultra soft, basic, chamomile, or sensitive? Hmmmmmmm. Hold on taco. Fine, I'll take the ultra strong for this taco. *What?* It's sold in a package of 4 or 6? I mean 4 or 6 or 8, 9, 12, 16, 18, 20, 24, 30, 36, 40, 45, or 48? I'll toss a coin. I mean I'll toss the cash register in front to decide. Seven coins, here it goes. Got it. I'll take the 24 pack. Ultra strong.

What? You must be kidding me. I've got 5 more choices—the mega, mega plus, double, double plus, or triple roll? You mean there are 70 combinations of ultra strong—5 roll types and 14 package sizes? Maybe I need the ultra soft after all. Only 56 combinations there. Wait, I've got my handy random number generator app since there are 149 different packages available in this brand across *toilet paper type*, *roll size*, and *package size* (so freaking annoying)! It's not like the 1970s when you had one type, one roll size, and one package size—it was so much easier wiping your ass back then! And no doubt when I *do* get home (tomorrow, since I'm still checking the toilet paper to be sure I got the right one), my wife is going to say I told you to get the *other* brand.

PA System—Clean up on Aisle Two!

I think I'm going to be sick. Where are the barf bags? They only come in one size right?

And *no*, the clean up on aisle two was *not* me.

Chapter 2

Buster, Neil, and Dan

In 2003, I purchased space to open a new office. The space was a shell, so I had to hire someone to do the upfit. I spoke with Curt White, a chiropractor who practiced adjacent to my office and found out that he had used Buster Williams of Southern Constructors to upfit his space. Curt spoke highly of Buster, so I decided that I would meet him. Buster came to my office on his Harley Davidson and looked like he was Jerry Garcia's brother. We spoke for a while, looked over my plans, and shortly thereafter he bid on my project. It would cost $200,000 to upfit my space. I considered having multiple contractors bid on the project but did not. While this seemed counter to common sense, I knew I didn't need any other bids. It's hard to put into words, but I *knew* Buster was the person to work with. A $200,000 project and I only needed one bid, Buster's.

From the outset, Buster was *always* looking out for me. Even before the upfit began in May of 2004, Buster advised me that the price of the metal studs needed for hanging drywall was going to be $8,000 if we waited to purchase them until May. However, if I purchased them in February, it was $5,000. Buster, tell me who to write out the check to for the $5,000. And so, right off the bat, Buster was looking out for me and saved me $3,000.

One of the things I remember most about Buster was a message he left on my home answering machine. His message said: "Doctor Wooooolfe........Buster......Southeeeerrnnnn." Buster's southern drawl was very characteristic. I loved it so much, I saved the message for weeks. I would replay it again and again. Buster's message was one of only two in my life I saved and replayed just to hear it again and again.

Doctor Woooolfe...........Doctor Woooolfe.............Doctor Woooolfe..............Buster...............Southeeeerrnnnnnn. Doctor Wooolfe.................Buster.............Southeeeerrnnnn. I played it every day for weeks. Usually the first thing I did when I got home from work was to play it. It made me smile.

Buster was honest and always looked out for me. Little did I know that he was moving a couple of hours away from Mooresville, North Carolina to Asheville, North Carolina. He had sold his home in Mooresville early on in the 100 or so days it took for my upfit. Unlike most people, he committed to my project and did it in earnest, delaying *his* move. He always put his customer first.

There are no words that can adequately describe Buster's genuineness, honesty, and character. I knew he was a gem the second I met him and every day I knew him. I believe if Buster recognized he had charged someone a penny too much for a project, he would have paid them $500 for the mistake. So for the largest project of my life I got to work with a construction and human saint. The project started *exactly* on time and ended *exactly* on time.

I also remember a story that Buster once told me. "Dr. Wolfe, I almost got a speeding ticket today." I asked him what happened. He said an officer pulled him over and said, "Do you know you were doing 45 in a 35 zone?" Buster's reply: "Wellllllllllll, that's a possibility." Did he get a ticket? Of course not. Buster was different in many ways.

Sadly, a couple of summers after my office was built, I learned of Buster's tragic and untimely death. He was up on a ladder at his home in Asheville and fell. During the fall, something punctured his femoral artery and he rapidly bled to death. I was devastated with the loss of such a great, kind, honest, and dedicated man. Someone whom I knew I could trust and whose character stood for itself. **I miss you Buster.**

While I only knew Buster for a relatively short time, the impact he had on my life was tremendous. I shall never forget Buster Williams. To this day, a decade or so later, I still find myself praying about him.

Now Neil, or Neil Platt, was my best friend for much of my elementary and middle school years. We grew up in Queens, New York. A lot of education and training took me far away from New York. A good 15 or 20 years after leaving New York, I called Neil and left him a message that I would be in New York and hoped we could get together.

He called me back and left a message on my answering machine. The same machine that had once stored Buster's message.

Steevin Wolfe..........Neil Platt...........New Yawk City. I loved this message so much that I kept it for a good month or so, just as I had kept Buster's. I played it every day. Steevin Wolfe...........Steevin Wolfe.............Steevin Wolfe...........Neil Platt..........New Yawk City. Neil Platt.........New Yawk City.

Steevin Wolfe...........Steevin Wolfe...........Neil Platt...........New Yawk City. I love ya Neil! You are one of only two people in my life whose message I kept for a month because I liked it.

Not to mention, when I did go to New York, Neil would always say the same thing. When I told him when and where I would be staying, he would say: "**I'll be there**." Once a great friend, always a great friend.

Dan. Well, he has a last name, but on the advice of an attorney he suggested not to mention his whole name. Dan had a plumbing company. The company would come out and either do a free or cheap whole house inspection. Then at the end they would find something that would be ridiculously expensive to fix.

One time, they told me my 1/2 bath toilet had a seal that didn't look good. In fact it needed to be fixed urgently. I needed a *toilet overhaul* (replace all the stuff in the tank). How much? $300. *What*, my toilet *isn't* leaking, but *migh*t leak in the future and I need to spend $300 to fix something that isn't broken? How much are the parts? $20?

Thanks for your advice. No thank you. I fixed it myself. Granted, not being a plumber, it took me 2 hours to do it but saved me $280. I was convinced that if I did the repair on another toilet I could do it in 30 minutes flat—pretty low learning curve! Besides, it doesn't even make sense to me today that if a seal is broken or eroding, why one has to replace *every* part inside the tank. Do you replace the engine in a car when the brakes aren't working?

About 15 years after I was almost ripped off, I ran into someone and told them this story. When I mentioned Dan, they amazingly had their *own* Dan story. They had avoided an $845 job that took $100 in parts and would have taken 30 minutes to fix. Once a crook, always a crook.

The moral of this chapter is that some people do things for you that cost *a lot of money*, yet they are completely honest and trustworthy. Character is something that is rare, and lasts a lifetime. Others are willing to rip you off for seemingly much smaller projects. I have found the world to be filled with a lot more of this type of person.

Character = **Rare**. Crook = **Common**.

For a link to see videos of Buster and Neil check
www.149waystowipeyourass.com/videos.html

Chapter 3

You Are A Wisenheimer

While I was a fourth year medical student doing a rotation at the VA Hospital in San Francisco, I had a rather elderly man as a patient. One day I was outside his room and was horsing around. He had obviously heard me.

As soon as I came in, the grandfatherly man blurted out, **"YOU ARE A WISENHEIMER!"** What made it even more interesting was his gravelly voice. To this day I don't recall how I responded. Perhaps if this was late night television I could have my top responses now.

1. Yes. Yes I am.

2. Well, that's a possibility. (Thanks Buster Williams)

3. That's **DOCTOR** Wisenheimer to you!

4. Once a Wisenheimer, always a Wisenheimer

5. Even though I want to be a doctor, I find it quite depressing to work in hospitals. I find humor one of

the few ways to get me through it. I find it keeps me sane, helping me to help you.

As an aside to #5, I still hate hospitals. Perhaps this is one of the reasons I became a dermatologist—my practice is virtually exclusively in the outpatient setting.

To see a video of the patient who called me a Wisenheimer go to

www.149waystowipeyourass.com/videos.html

Chapter 4

The Book of Excuses

A few summers ago, I hired someone to do some repairs on my pontoon boat. I asked him how long it would take to fix. He told me it would be fixed in two weeks. Well, two weeks passed and it wasn't fixed. He had gotten called out of town unexpectedly.

Three weeks passed and it wasn't fixed. He was waiting on a part. Four weeks passed and it wasn't fixed. His partner had quit.

Five weeks passed and it wasn't fixed. He had a kidney stone. Six weeks passed and it wasn't fixed. His truck had a flat tire. So I called him.

ME: "Johnson........is my boat fixed?"

JOHNSON: "I should have it back next week. My bathroom flooded and the repair guys have been here all week."

ME: "Johnson......have you read the book?"

JOHNSON: "The book?"

ME: "Yeah, the book."

JOHNSON: "What book?"

ME: "THE BOOK OF EXCUSES!!!! BECAUSE YOU'VE GIVEN ME EVERY ONE!!!!!!!!"

Chapter 5

The Book of Excuses, Part II

This chapter might hurt the sales of my book, but even if it does, too bad. So before you read further, if you work in I/T, you might want to skip to the next chapter without reading this one.

I'm a dermatologist and more than 10 years ago my group, along with many practices in the United States, converted to Electronic Medical Records (EMR). I, along with most of the other 1,000,000 doctors in the United States, would likely agree this was a critical step in the demise of practicing medicine. It was supposed to increase efficiency, allow you to see more patients, and increase revenues. Well, is the *Pope* Jewish?

A little digression. Two thousand five hundred ninety-seven is the record for strikeouts by a batter in the major leagues. Presumably, being the all time leader for striking out at bat is not a title you want to have. This batter, however, did hit 563 home runs in his career and he was quite popular and an amazing player. I still remember him well and loved watching him play. (Reggie Jackson).

A prior head of our I/T department, who we'll call **"STRIKEOUT,"** in my opinion *never* hit a home run. Being the New Yorker that I am, I have a way of telling it like it is. No reason to sugar coat things. I recall an email I sent to **STRIKEOUT**.

> *From: Doctor Wolfe@Iamafunnydoctor.com*
> *To: **STRIKEOUT**@yourI/Tservicesucks.com*
> *Subject: Crash*
>
> ***STRIKEOUT,***
>
> *Our computers crash more than a stock car in the Daytona 500 driven by a one armed driver who just underwent cataract surgery and when they do run, they are slower than a stock car with a blown engine.*
>
> *Now seriously, it is no more fun for me to send these emails than it is for you to receive them........*
>
> *Dr. Wolfe*

Suffice it to say, **STRIKEOUT** did not appreciate my sense of humor.

STRIKEOUT would use all sorts of euphemisms about the I/T problems our group had. He would write emails saying that the system was like an onion........it had a lot of layers. The only thing that I agreed with regarding this analogy was that the whole system stunk *and* made me cry.

Now back to the *Book of Excuses*. One time the whole system went down. **STRIKEOUT** explained the "downtime."

This is from his actual email:

1. A storm hit the area creating a power outage.

2. The generator did not start.

3. The batteries on the UPS in the data center drained.

4. The data center went dark.

Later in his explanation he noted that the generator had a dead battery and a fried charger. The charger had shorted due to rats chewing the cables. The battery, which was only two months old, was being replaced with a new one. Things would be functional as soon as they got all the parts in the generator.

A year after **STRIKEOUT** was "no longer employed by our organization" things didn't really improve. Each time some disaster occurred, we got another email from the *I/T Book Of Excuses*.

Over a period of 10 years I can best summarize things as follows: our computers and I/T needs are as reliable as having unprotected sex in Africa with a prostitute and hoping not to contract an STD. And as far as electronic medical records making you faster, the only thing it will make you do faster is *retire*.

Chapter 6

Do You Like My Hair?
The Toilet is Clogged

I've been married now for 23 years and known my wife for 25 years. Sometimes I get home and I see that she has gotten her hair cut and colored. As soon as I get home I notice it and think it looks *really* good and that's exactly what I'm about to tell her. Just before I say this, she tells me that the toilet is clogged in the downstairs bathroom. So I check out the toilet. When I'm lucky, it's clogged and the water level is low. When I'm unlucky, it's clogged and the water level is high. If I'm really unlucky, it's clogged, the water level is high, and (this might be more information than you wanted, so I'm going to leave it at that).

I go get the gloves and the plunger. Sometimes it's a few plunges, other times a bunch. When it's a really bad day you get plunger elbow. OK, finally, got it. Unclogged. So I head back to the kitchen to be with my wife.

First thing she says: "You didn't comment about my hair!"

I respond: "Well, I noticed it as soon as I came in the door and the first words out of my mouth were about to be, gee, you got your hair cut and colored and it looks *really* good, but you threw me the toilet is clogged before I could say anything. By the time I got the toilet unclogged, it just slipped my mind."

I hope there are some husbands out there who know this scenario and I hope my wife doesn't read this chapter.

Chapter 7

SMOOT

Back in the 1980s, there was a skit on Saturday Night Live called Dick Clark's Receptionist. David Spade played the receptionist. A variety of famous people would enter the office and would be greeted by David Spade. In a rather drawn out and obnoxious way he would say: "And you are? And this is regarding?"

A few examples of guests who walked in included MC Hammer, Roseanne Arnold, and Jesus. Of course it would particularly incense these famous people not to be recognized or acknowledged.

A few years later, I was doing my medical internship at UCLA. It was 1992. In my second month of internship I had a rotation at the VA Hospital in West Los Angeles. My rotation was in the ICU (intensive care unit) and my resident on this rotation was Dr. Craig Mitchell. Oh, and by the way, Dr. Mitchell was a fan of Saturday Night Live.

One night (it seemed that everything happened at night when I was an intern) a patient came in who was gorked out (mentally out of it). It was a little after midnight. The gentleman's last name was Smoot. Smoot was relatively alert, but definitely not oriented. His family recognized a fairly sudden and dramatic change of mental status in Mr. Smoot and appropriately brought him to the hospital. Mr. Smoot was about 70 years old.

Being at the VA hospital, the residents and interns had to do almost everything. We were not only physicians, we had to do things that most other hospitals had ancillary staff to do, like draw blood and wheel patients to get CT scans. So Dr. Mitchell and I went into action. A sudden change of mental status can be a harbinger of many serious underlying conditions. Amongst other things, altered mental status can result from intoxication, endocrine abnormalities, abnormal electrolytes, encephalopathy, infection, kidney failure, trauma, poisoning, psychiatric disturbance, strokes, and tumors.

These conditions, if not recognized and treated quickly, could result in the death of a patient, so we worked quickly to try and establish a diagnosis and intervene. We ordered a variety of blood tests, did blood cultures, a urine culture, ordered a chest x-ray, got an EKG, did a lumbar puncture and arranged for a CT scan to exclude a stroke or brain tumor. We immediately started antibiotics since things such as meningitis, encephalitis, sepsis, septic shock, pneumonia and urinary tract infections can cause altered mental status. Given the circumstances, it was better to institute therapies that weren't needed but would likely have little risk, than to withhold treatments until we had a final answer only to realize that the delay resulted in the death of the patient whom we were trying to save.

We had already sent off the blood tests and cultures and

were awaiting the lumbar puncture results. We also had the results of the chest x-ray which excluded pneumonia and the EKG was normal. Next up, Dr. Mitchell and I functioned as orderlies and had to get Mr. Smoot to the CT scanner to exclude stroke or other brain abnormality. By now it was after 2 a.m. and we had been attending to Mr. Smoot for a good hour and a half. We wheeled Mr. Smoot through the halls to the elevator.

Once on the elevator, Dr. Mitchell turned to our patient and reminiscent of Saturday Night Live, said to him in a slowly spoken manner: "And you are?"

Almost instantly our patient who was mentally out of it said: "SMOOT."

Dr. Mitchell continued, "And this is regarding?"

I don't think SMOOT had an answer for that one, though he may have just repeated again, "SMOOT."

As the elevator got us to the right level and we wheeled Mr. Smoot quickly to the CT scanning room, Dr. Mitchell would occasionally repeat his same inquiry. "And you are?"

Each time, Mr. Smoot would respond, "SMOOT."

Essentially this accomplished the mental status exam along the way to the CT scanner. Smoot was oriented to person, but not to place and time.

The CT scan excluded a stroke or brain tumor. The blood tests excluded most common things such as electrolyte abnormalities, endocrine abnormalities and kidney failure. The blood cultures we had drawn, looking for an infection, would take a day or two to come back. By now it was almost 4 a.m. We had done everything we could to exclude most of the medical emergencies off our list, but still could not exclude infection. A few short hours later, when we were doing rounds in the morning, we came to Mr. Smoot's room in the ICU. He was *completely* lucid.

As it turned out, Mr. Smoot had been in his garage a day or two earlier and gotten a small cut on his leg. That cut had introduced an infection into his blood stream causing his change of mental status. His resulting sepsis would have resulted in septic shock and death if not treated. Fortunately, the antibiotics we had immediately started saved Mr. Smoot's life. I'd estimate he would have succumbed within a day or two if we hadn't treated him.

Dr. Mitchell and I have remained friends over the last 23 years and we never forget the night we saw and saved Mr. Smoot. We also never forget our Saturday Night Live skit that provided a little humor and energy to sustain us during those long hours of the night.

Twenty-three years later, Dr. Mitchell and I often still start our conversations with the word SMOOT or the phrase: *"And you are?"*

Chapter 8

Weiners

...I've had to examine more than a few as a dermatologist...

Sometime back, a politician left himself exposed to a lot of humor. Of course this predicament happened because he had literally left himself exposed. His name didn't help matters either.

When this scandal broke, I had been a dermatologist for 12 years. An observation that I had made in practice was that if a male recognized *any* abnormality on his private parts it was certainly going to be brought to my attention.

So when this political scandal broke, I considered myself an expert on male anatomy and its problems and figured I should chime in with my own thoughts. Of course I've never understood how someone can think that they can text a (naked) picture, or email something, or be in a room where anyone has a cell phone, or post something on Facebook, and not have something come back to haunt them.

Getting back to the matter at hand, WEINER, here's what I came up with.

- ♂ Just in, WEINER cut off by family.
- ♂ Just in, Gag order issued at WEINER trial.
- ♂ Representative WEINER's son, Frank, stepson, Wong, first cousin, Peter, co-representative, Johnson, and urologist, I.M. Hung, report that they are dismayed with WEINER's actions.
- ♂ WEINER has taken a job with the FBI as an undercover agent and promises to be an upstanding member.
- ♂ WEINER's car broke down, but Pelosi said she'd be happy to take him for a ride.
- ♂ Pelosi was asked how she got WEINER to resign. She said, "I've been on top of WEINER since the first photo was released." In fact, she said she really, really liked WEINER, but unfortunately, he had become a distraction.
- ♂ Pelosi was asked if she saw WEINER leaving Congress. She said she saw him slip out the back door.
- ♂ When asked about her influence on WEINER's resignation, Pelosi said, "I had WEINER in the palm of my hand."
- ♂ Yesterday, at the gas station, Pelosi was in a car wreck with WEINER. After filling up, she hit the gas and backed into WEINER. No injuries were initially reported, but she notes she is a little sore today.
- ♂ The electricity was shut off at WEINER's house. This makes for one hot WEINER.
- ♂ WEINER, you seem down.
- ♂ Ex Cheers star, Shelley Long, has confessed that she and Congressman WEINER not only had an affair, but they are engaged to be married. Regarding WEINER's current state of affairs and possible criminal charges, the future

Mrs. Long-WEINER said, "If the glove don't fit, you must acquit."

♂ WEINER staying out of public eye.

♂ WEINER's wife tells WEINER it's time for a sit down.

♂ Police throw the book at WEINER and it bounces off.

♂ NBC Announces its fall lineup. Its newest show, The Biggest WEINER.

♂ And lastly, WEINER's wife tells WEINER to beat it.

Chapter 9

TJ Swift
(Kick in Your Ass)

I went to college at Case Western Reserve University in Cleveland, Ohio where I majored in chemistry and economics. One of my chemistry professors was TJ Swift. Professor Swift was not a big man, but it looked like he could do some damage if you got on his wrong side. I remember one day during a chemistry lecture someone was horsing around towards the back of a rather large lecture hall. Swift stopped the lecture and slowly, but deliberately walked up the stairs one at a time until he got to the row of the offender. The best that I can recall is that he told the person to get up and leave. It didn't appear that the matter was up for debate. I don't recall Swift yelling, cursing, or doing anything physical. He made his point and the screwball in the lecture hall got the message. Perhaps TJ did turn a little red.

TJ reminds me of a small number of highly regimented professors and teachers I had along the way. There was Mr.

Seibel in math class in 7th or 8th grade. An infraction with Seibel spelled the famous exercise of writing at least 100 times the thing you did and should not have done. I recall Mr. Rocco in 7th grade music class. He was lean, fit, and bald, like the Mr. Clean guy. One day Richard Rosenberg wasn't paying attention in class. Immediately, Rocco said: "Richard, if you don't stop messing around, I'll use that clarinet as a rectal thermometer." I guarantee nobody in class wanted to cross Rocco again.

I must confess, I did once get on Rocco's bad side, but not too bad. I played clarinet and hated it. I wanted to play the drums. So one time when Rocco was out sick I did play them. I don't know how he found out, but I remember the 200 or 300 times I had to write "I must not play the drums when Mr. Rocco is out sick." It was well worth it for getting to play the drums.

I recall Mr. Bursky in high school history class. He also didn't like people who didn't pay attention and like TJ, he didn't seem to be someone you wanted to cross. One day a girl was laughing in class. Bursky stopped the class and walked up the aisle. This did not look good.

He turned to her and in a snide way said, "If there's something so funny why don't you share it with us? We could all use a good laugh."

TJ, Seibel, Rocco and Bursky all shared the same thing. They did not put up with bullshit.

Similarly, I recall an attending physician at the VA hospital in West Los Angeles who would say rounds begin at 9 a.m., not 9:01 a.m. This kind of expectation seemed easy. The professor, instructor, teacher, or attending physician told you just what they expected. So do what they expect and everything works fine. It never made sense to me why anyone would have a problem with this type of personality. Do it this way and everything will be fine. Cross me and it won't. TJ, Seibel, Rocco, Bursky and that attending physician all made their expectations evidently clear so it was actually simple to be on their good side.

So why did I name this chapter after TJ Swift? Because one thing more than any other stands out to me about him. On his tests there would often be a question that required working through *a lot* of calculations.

A great deal of chemistry is like this. For instance you are given a solution that's an acid. You have to figure out the strength of the acid. To do so, you'll have to measure a powder that's a base. You'll have to dissolve it in a measured volume of liquid. Then you'll have to titrate carefully until you neutralize the acid. You have to measure everything carefully—weights and volumes. If you screw up one measurement, all of your calculations will be off and your final answer will be further from the true answer. This is especially true if you screw something up at the beginning.

The test question worked similarly. You had to do one calculation that led to another and then another and then another and finally you got the answer. TJ was a pretty straightforward guy. It all came down to the final answer.

Right = full credit. Wrong = no credit.

Typically the question was worth 10 or 20% of the whole test, so if you didn't get the FINAL answer right, boom, you're penalized 10 or 20%, a big hunk of the test. Most students were livid about this. They would argue that they should get partial credit, since 4 out of 5 of their calculations were correct. For TJ, life was a 5 out of 5 or nothing type of game.

We live in a world where too many people think in terms of partial credit. Would you like the engine of your car to be built 100% correct or 99% correct? Should the steering wheel be attached 98.5% tight or 100% tight? When I remove your skin cancer should I strive for 100% perfect or is 97% ok? When the pilot is flying your 737 home, is it ok to estimate the landing approach 98% correct? TJ drove this point home when a college student should recognize that correct = correct and wrong = wrong.

Thank you TJ. I always did, and still do respect you for the standards you had. A valuable lesson.

Chapter 10

Seymour Butts' Temporary Cure for Alzheimer's

Fred was a patient of mine in his mid 70s. He was a talented musician amongst other things, at least until his memory started failing. I had the pleasure of taking care of him for 5 or 6 years. As Fred's Alzheimer's disease worsened, he became more and more agitated. I've found that in my two decades of practicing medicine, people who are agitated usually also make me feel agitated. I'm no psychologist, but I'd say it's because I'm aware they are agitated, would like to fix it, but often cannot. So the agitation remains during their whole visit. It's not like someone who comes in worried that the benign spot they have is cancer and all you have to do is reassure them that it is not cancer.

I was aware of at least one thing that made Fred agitated and that was finances. He always complained that the place he lived cost so much. If I approached things with logic and asked if he had enough money (which I believe he did), that didn't seem to alleviate things. Likewise, if I touched upon the idea that the only consequence might be his children having a smaller inheritance, that didn't seem to reduce Fred's agitation either. It even failed if I took the most obvious approach, namely asking Fred if he liked where he lived.

Seemingly, the thing that agitated Fred the most was really rather simple. I could see his cogs turning, but they just wouldn't turn the right way for Fred to get out what he was struggling to. I think he was keenly aware of this disability and it appeared to both annoy and agitate him. I truly wished I could fix it. One day, at least for a little while, I did.

In my office, I have been known to hand out all kinds of goodies to patients. During my entire career I've given out Dum Dums lollipops. In fact, this has become such a ritual that the 1% or less of the time I forget to do it, whoever I am seeing says: "Where's my Dum Dums lollipop?" I immediately apologize that I forgot to give them one and produce one out of my pocket. Sometimes I produce two because I forgot to give them one. Early on in practice, not only did I give out Dum Dums lollipops, I did magic tricks for patients. As my practice got busier though, I didn't have time to do that and had to stop.

I've also given out other forms of candy, lighted suckers, chocolate cigars, fake cigars, fake cigarettes, tattoo sleeves, fake diamond earrings, t-shirts, baseball caps, bandanas, denim jackets, sweatshirts, can holders, zip-up bottle holders, stuffed animals, stickers, voodoo dolls, whoopee cushions, fart putty, pieces of art, cookie cutters, ice-packs, laughing head pens, relax/calm down pens, popping eyeball pens, spacey eyeglasses, rainbow goo-goo eyeglasses, eyebrow and moustache eyeglasses, nerd eyeglasses, bouncing balls, stick to the wall toys, Laphroaig Single Malt Scotch (Jim Diers) and one of my very favorite things—5" X 7" photos that are in a folder display. These are *always* photos that I have taken, often on my travels. Many times I just give out a cool photo of a penguin, or a Sally Lightfoot Crab, or a sunset to a patient. Sometimes a specific photo comes to mind based on the patient and circumstances that present. That's what happened with Fred.

Now about a year before this one particular visit with Fred, I was at a very important dermatology conference in Aruba. Certainly, any dermatology conference in Aruba is very important. Namely, very important that I get to tax deduct the trip and *go* to Aruba.

While there, in addition to attending the conference, I had some time to stay on the beach (with sunscreen and sun protective clothing and a hat). I also had my camera and my favorite lens, a 70-300 mm lens. This allowed me to get photos from far away and have them look like I was right next to the subject. In addition to taking photographs I wanted to practice my power to predict the future. Sometimes I was *really* good at predicting the future. In Aruba, I was *excellent.*

Here's what I would do. I would look down the beach and watch people who were far away walking *towards* me. I must confess, this was always women unless they were with their partner. My goal was to predict which of these women in bikinis had the type of bikini that has virtually no material on the backside. I found that I was *very* good at this exercise. Once said subject passed me, the 70-300 mm lens took care of all of the rest. One particular photo I cropped just perfectly. It was a near perfect shot of a female behind. This shot has made many, many people very happy.

Back to Fred. I had my doubts about giving this photo to Fred. Before I seriously entertained the idea, I said to myself,

"What kind of doctor does such a thing?" My photos are stored in my back office, so when I decide to give one to someone, I leave the exam room and return with it.

Fred's cogs weren't turning so well, but mine were. I had it all figured out even if I didn't know exactly what was going to happen. I told Fred I'd be back in a minute. I left and went to the back and returned with the photo in a folder labeled *Beach babe's buttock*. I didn't immediately give it to Fred.

Instead, I said to Fred that I knew he was concerned about his memory loss. I knew this got him down. But I said to Fred that I thought his memory was in fact far better than he thought. He didn't quite know what I meant. Then, I produced the photo folder and opened it. Fred had a *very, very* big smile on his face.

That's when I told Fred, "See Fred, your memory *is* better than you think."

Some things you never forget. At that point of the visit, I can testify that Fred's agitation had completely gone away, at least for a time. I knew I had done my job. God Bless You Fred.

See the photo I showed Fred on my website:
www.149waystowipeyourass.com/images

Chapter 11

Mr. Whalley, OK, OK

Having practiced medicine for nearly 20 years, I've had just shy of 100,000 separate patient encounters. Some of my favorites were with a patient named Mr. Whalley.

When I first met Mr. Whalley, I recall entering the exam room at his first visit, introducing myself, and asking him how he was doing. He replied, "OK, OK." Mr. Whalley was a short man, a little overweight, and was a retired postal worker. He was 87 when I first met him. His favorite hobby was fishing. That was good for me and bad for him. The more YOU are in the sun, the more skin problems, a good thing for me professionally. Mr. Whalley had moved down from Long Island, New York to North Carolina to be closer to family. He had a boat when he lived on Long Island, so his prior sun exposure resulted in his needing frequent visits to see me.

Back to the OK, OK. When I asked Mr. Whalley how he was doing and he told me "OK, OK." He said it in a very calm, comforting, easy going way. He struck me as a kind, pleasant, soft spoken and relaxed man. In fact, every time he came to see me, I'd ask him how he was doing, and he was always positive and calming and said the same thing, "OK, OK."

So even when my day had sucked, getting to see Mr. Whalley always made my day better. Just seeing his name on my schedule made me feel happy. Mr. Whalley was "OK , OK," and suddenly I was too.

At the age of 87, I am sure Mr. Whalley faced a variety of challenges, but he was always positive, calming, and made me feel better just getting to see him. I felt very connected to Mr. Whalley. So much so, that three years after meeting him, when he was turning 90, he invited me to his 90th birthday party. I would not miss it for anything.

For his birthday, I painted a 24 inch square canvas with a red, white, and blue heart. It was a very calming piece of art. As calming as seeing and taking care of Mr. Whalley. It was a blessing to attend his 90th birthday party and be a part of such a momentous day in this lovely man's life. Today, the day I am writing this, is 3 days short of the 8-year anniversary of that day, July 13, 2007.

Very shortly after turning 90, Mr. Whalley fell and broke his hip. With his advanced age and underlying health conditions, this was very serious. I received a call from Mr. Whalley's family that he was in the hospital and having a lot of complications. They did not expect him to survive. Knowing that I was very close to him they wanted me to know in case I wanted to see him.

Later that day I went to the hospital to visit Mr. Whalley. He was asleep in bed. He seemed so peaceful, so much so that I had to think hard about whether or not I should wake him up to speak with him. After a few minutes, I decided I would. I wanted him to know that I was there.

So I gently rubbed his shoulder until he opened his eyes and I said, "Mr. Whalley, it's Doctor Wolfe. How are you doing?"

Mr. Whalley said exactly the same thing he told me every time I had seen him in the three years I knew him. "OK, OK."

The next day Mr. Whalley passed away. I was so fortunate to have been blessed with the opportunity to take care of such a wonderful, kind, and calming man. Mr. Whalley was short in stature and tall in character and kindness. It was very emotional, yet cathartic to write this. I think Mr. Whalley contradicts the non-calming nature of our world. I truly bawled just writing this, particularly the part that even when my day sucked, Mr. Whalley always made it better for me, seemingly without even trying.

I hope I made your days better too Mr. Whalley.

For a link to a video in tribute to Mr. Whalley see
www.149waystowipeyourass.com/videos.html

Chapter 12

Mom's Tomato Sauce

Shortly after I finished dermatology training, we moved to Greensboro, North Carolina. The year was 1996. There was a very nice, small, upscale market very close to the house we were renting. One time my wife went shopping there and bought a jar of tomato sauce. The sauce happened to be named Mom's. It had fresh whole garlic cloves, whole basil leaves and beautiful tomatoes.

My wife made spaghetti one night and served it with Mom's Tomato Sauce. *Wow*! It was *really* good! It was one of the best sauces I had ever tasted. After I finished eating, I was curious and asked her how much Mom's cost. She said she hadn't checked the price.

So I pulled it out of the garbage to see if it had a price sticker on it. It did. It was $5.99. Now this was back at a time when there weren't 47 brands of tomato sauce and chefs with funny clogs or yelling **BAM** at you who had their own brand of tomato sauce. Likewise, it was at a time when most jars of tomato sauce cost $2. Finally, it was at a time that I still had

$41,000 of medical school debt to pay back. So $5.99 was a lot of money.

I'm sure my wife could probably recite the rest of this conversation, even now, almost 20 years later. It probably went something like this, **"What!** You spent $5.99 on a jar of *tomato sauce* and you didn't even *know* it cost $5.99!" This is another chapter that I hope my wife doesn't read. In her defense, though, it was the best sauce we had ever eaten.

I do not consider myself a cheapskate. However, I believe strongly in value. You have to know that what you are getting is worth what you are paying. A high risk situation is when you don't know what you are paying. Over the years I can recall a variety of price mistakes that my wife or I have made. The *glass* of wine in the late 1990s that cost $27, at a time when you could buy a nice *bottle* for less. The time on the cruise that the bottle of wine cost $135 (we usually spent $30 for a bottle). And, sadly, the two glasses of champagne we drank at lunch at a famous Italian chef's New York City restaurant costing us $50 for *each* glass. All of those circumstances shared one thing in common. We did not know the price of the thing we were buying, nor were we told.

My way of thinking in the past was simple, but wrong. My old way of thinking was that *you*, the server, should tell someone like *me*, the customer, if something is stupid expensive. Unfortunately, that's not the way it works. Particularly for glasses of wine, single malt scotches, and specials of the day. Some might say if you have to ask, you can't afford it. Usually, I *can* afford it, I just don't think it's worth it and I'd like to be given the option of turning down something that's ridiculously overpriced. Fortunately, asking, "How much?" has saved us from a lot more costly mistakes than those we have made. It is better to be informed than to be surprised.

Since we are on the topic of food, I have another scenario for discontent. This is when you *do* know what you are paying. Restaurants that cost six times the amount we usually spend never make me feel six times better than ones that cost 1/6 as much. I'd name some of the famous chefs who owned the restaurants where we made these 6X as much as we usually spend mistakes, but those famous chefs have a lot more money than I do and I don't want any trouble. I try to follow my 3X rule. Never spend more than 3X the amount you commonly spend on a meal. It's never worth it. *Buon appetito!*

Chapter 13

Chan: What? No Tip!

Back in 2005, my friend, Dr. Craig Mitchell (the doctor who worked with me at the West Los Angeles VA Hospital and undeniably saved Mr. Smoot's life), got married in Las Vegas.

While we were there, he said, "Hey, why don't we take a limousine to go somewhere?" So we did.

That somewhere was maybe a mile from where we were. When we got there, our driver, Chan, told us it was $50. We were stunned, but what could we do? So we each tossed in $5 or $10 until we had the $50 and reluctantly we gave it to Chan.

He counted it, looked at us, and then said, "WHAT, NO TIP?"

We didn't give him a tip, but that remark was enough to keep Dr. Mitchell and me creating humor for weeks.

Every time we spoke, we'd say, "Chan, What? No Tip!" One or the other of us had a new remark almost daily for weeks.

These are some of our all time favorites and they always start the same way.

Chan, What? No Tip!
Chan, you want a tip?

Here's your tip: Next time you drive us a mile, only charge us $40 and we'll give you a tip!

Chan, What? No Tip!
Chan, you want a tip?

Here's your tip: If you charged us $50 to go to the airport, instead of across the street, we would have given you a tip!

Chan, What? No Tip!
Chan, you want a tip?

Here's your tip: Work in a restaurant if you want to get a tip!

Chan, What? No Tip!
Chan, you want a tip?

Here's your tip: It is better to get in a buffet line before someone who is morbidly obese instead of after them!

Chan, What? No Tip!
Chan, you want a tip?

Here's your tip: If they are calling for rain, be sure to close your moon roof!

Chan, What? No Tip!
Chan, you want a tip?

Here's your tip: Don't forget to tighten the nuts
after you change a tire!

Chan, What? No Tip!
Chan, you want a tip?

Here's a tip: The term smokin', when referring to
a chick, is good. The term smokin', when referring
to your limousine, is bad.

Chan, What? No Tip!
Chan, you want a tip?

Here's your tip: When Rodney King asked, "Can't
we all just get along?" The answer was NO!

Chan, What? No Tip!
Chan, you want a tip?

Here's your tip: When your wife says, "If I buy this
(whatever it is) I'll never need another one," don't
believe her!

Chan, What? No Tip!
Chan, you want a tip?

Here's your tip: Remember the hot chick at the
bar who said she'll call you? She was lying!

Chan, What? No Tip!
Chan, you want a tip?

Here's your tip: Be sure you have nickels, dimes, and quarters when you get into the exact change toll lane!

Chan, What? No Tip!
Chan, you want a tip?

Here's your tip: Don't play golf in the rain!

Chan, What? No Tip!
Chan, you want a tip?

Here's your tip: Don't iron your clothes while wearing them!

Chan, What? No Tip!
Chan, you want a tip?

Here's your tip: Don't lick dry ice!

Chan, What? No Tip!
Chan, you want a tip?

Here's your tip: Always wear shoes in a dog park!

Chan, What? No Tip!
Chan, you want a tip?

Here's your tip: If you are an operator at the suicide hotline, never say, "Can you hold, please?"

Chan, What? No Tip!
Chan, you want a tip?

Here's your tip: Don't eat onions on a first date if you want to have a second date!

Chan, What? No Tip!
Chan, you want a tip?

Here's your tip: When your girlfriend says, "It's not you, it's me", it *IS* you!

Chan, What? No Tip!
Chan, you want a tip?

Here's your tip: When your girlfriend says, "Let's just be friends," she means, "I never want to see you again!"

Chan, What? No Tip!
Chan, you want a tip?

Here's your tip: Don't kiss your girlfriend when she has a fever blister!

Chan, What? No Tip!
Chan, you want a tip?

When you go to the bathroom, *always* check for toilet paper *before* you sit down.

While I've tried to generally stay away from relationship and marital advice in this book, I decided to put in one last piece of advice as it seemed apropos in this chapter.

Chan, What? No Tip!
Chan, you want a tip?

Here's your tip: The three worst words you can
hear from a woman you are in a relationship with
are, "CAN WE TALK?"

Still to this day, when my friend Craig and I speak, we often throw in a Chan, What? No Tip!

The moral of this story? That $50 fare to travel one mile in Las Vegas actually took us a whole lot farther than we thought.

Part II

How S&M, A Free Ticket to California
And My 30 Days of Addiction
Led Me To Become A Dermatologist

Chapter 14

I've Loved S&M For a Long Time

Before we get into some S&M, let me give you some background. It is often said that the S.T.E.M. fields hold the most promise for advancement both on an individual basis and for our country. S.T.E.M. stands for science, technology, engineering, and mathematics. I have always been fascinated by S&M, that is, science and mathematics.

I was fortunate to have many great science and math teachers, particularly in high school. One teacher, Mr. Morton Roggen, encouraged me to do special science programs during the summer. These were held at a few universities across the United States. I was able to participate in one program at Michigan State University after my sophomore year in high school and another at Indiana University after my junior year in high school. I had the opportunity to participate in some interesting research projects while there. Though I had little real exposure to medicine *per se* at that time, my love of science was enough to make me think that a career in medicine might be the right choice for me.

Although I didn't have an exact plan in mind, this was the reason I looked at colleges that had combined college/medical school programs. Some of these programs accelerated your education, letting you skip one and sometimes even two years of college. I did not want to skip any years of college so I only looked at programs that did not require you to accelerate your education.

While I was applying to these combined college/medical school programs it was my belief that it would take the pressure off of having to apply to medical school. If medical school was the right thing, I would have a secure spot. I also felt this would allow me more freedom to pursue studies and experiences that I otherwise might not pursue if I had to apply to medical school the old fashioned way. This alone, made Case Western Reserve University a good choice for me. The other part of my decision was financial. I wanted a free college education.

Chapter 15

The $34,000 Essay (1984)

In 1984, I applied to a dozen or so colleges. One of them was Case Western Reserve University (CWRU). CWRU was one of the only colleges in the United States that offered an academic full tuition scholarship *and* an 8-year combined college and medical school program that guaranteed you a slot into their medical school even before *starting* college. Of course there were a few contingencies on this acceptance to medical school. You had to have a minimum 3.4 GPA (rather low compared to what you would need applying to medical school as a college senior) and you could not receive less than a "B" in any of the important classes (Chemistry, Biology, Organic Chemistry and the like). I was accepted into the medical program. So I knew I had a guaranteed spot into medical school. All I had to do was 4 years of college and meet the minimum GPA requirement and get a B or higher in the important stuff.

The full tuition scholarship was of course based on grades, SAT scores, letters of recommendation and extracurricular activities. I had that part handled with no problems. The last part was that you had to write an essay while at their campus. Presumably, this was the only thing keeping me from the full tuition scholarship.

The essay topic was, "Do grades predict success?" I broke my answer into four parts.

1. Some people get bad grades, but they are actually geniuses. Often, these people don't apply themselves, but as noted, they are very smart. I think some of them do end up being successful. Perhaps the only thing keeping them from success is themselves. It is of course a shame to waste a great mind, but many do.

2. Some people get bad grades and they in fact are not very smart. I think that they generally end up not being successful. Though of course it depends on how you define success. If you define it as some type of job or career that requires lots of education, this type of person probably does reach a dead end.

3. Some people get great grades, yet are not successful. Some of these people of course get great grades by cheating. Sooner or later, that is likely to catch up with them. Other people get great grades, but they have no common sense. Common sense is an important attribute to have in order to be successful. So if you are a cheater, or pretty smart, but have no common sense, your level of success could be far lower than your grades predict.

4. Some people get good grades, get them honestly, and do have common sense. They also apply themselves. I think this group excels the most in our society.

The moral of the story, and the crux of my answer, was that sometimes grades *do* predict success and sometimes they *don't.*

Fortunately, I got the full tuition scholarship. It was worth $34,000 for my four years of college tuition between 1984 and 1988. Thank you CWRU for allowing me to have a free college education and allowing me to graduate with no undergraduate debt. Most of all, thank you for guaranteeing me a slot into medical school. This took the pressure off and allowed me to do many things that most premeds would never do. Going to London for my junior year was just one of those things.

Chapter 16

Blood Dripping Onto The Floor

It was June 9, 1986. I had recently turned 20 years old and finished my sophomore year of college. I applied and was accepted into a program at Cleveland Metro General Hospital that's called the Chester Summer Scholars Program. At 8 a.m. I arrived at Dr. Gerding's office. He was my sponsor for the summer and I was eager to find out what awaited. When I arrived, I found a closed door. I searched until I found Dr. Gerding's secretary who told me that Dr. Gerding was in the operating room (OR) and would not be out before noon. I dejectedly walked back to my room at the dormitory of the hospital and waited. At about 10 a.m. I received a phone call. It was Dr. Gerding's secretary. She said that Dr. Gerding wanted to see me immediately—IN THE OPERATING ROOM!

Shortly after I arrived, a rather young, friendly doctor emerged through a set of electronically operated doors. It was Dr. Gerding.

After introducing himself he said, "This summer is for you

and the most important thing is to enjoy yourself. I am taking you into the OR because seeing an operation, specifically a burn operation, will allow you to understand the importance of the research project that you will be working on."

As I changed into surgical scrubs, Dr. Gerding described Gary Williams, the patient they were operating on. Gary was 36 and had burns, mostly second and third degree, covering some 50% of his body. Dr. Gerding explained that burn surgery tended to be bloody and if I felt uneasy in the OR I should not be embarrassed—we would leave. When I finished changing, Dr. Gerding asked if I was ready. My reply was an emphatic "Yes!".

When we entered the OR, the chief resident was directing the operation. He was removing burnt tissue from Mr. Williams' back. As he and the junior residents removed tissue, Gary began to bleed. During this procedure two things disturbed me. First, the radio was on. How could they listen to the radio during such a serious operation? The second thing that disturbed me was the blood dripping onto the floor. Weren't they going to stop the bleeding?

No sooner than I thought of this, the chief resident applied electrocautery to the places that were bleeding the most profusely. Suddenly, the radio developed static as the smell of burning human flesh permeated the air. How paradoxical to be treating a burn with yet another burn.

Wait. I was beginning to understand. The radio was there to relieve tension and make the doctors and nurses feel more relaxed. Of course. Could it be any other way? As for the bleeding and burning flesh, they were both part of the treatment required to save Gary's life. What an experience to be watching an operation in progress. I wondered if I would become a surgeon.

That afternoon, Dr. Gerding and I went to see Mr. Williams. He was in pain, but his spirits were high considering what he had been through. Dr. Gerding treated Gary on a personal level. In addition, he considered Gary's family. He said things that comforted Gary's family such as, "Gary is a fighter and he is going to make it."

"But how could they manage with Gary out of work and with the hospital bills?" they asked.

Dr. Gerding told them that the insurance coverage Gary's employer had (Gary was burned while working at a silk-screening plant) would cover all of the medical bills. And, in a few months, Gary would be able to go back to work.

"In the meantime," he said, "Gary needs support. He needs a positive self-image and you can all help him." Once again, Dr. Gerding assured them that Gary was doing well and they would be able to see him that afternoon.

Now Gary's family was a picture of joy relative to their appearance only minutes before. The tragedy still existed, but Gary was receiving the best care available. Dr. Gerding showed me the importance of dealing with the patient and their family. In short, he taught me the importance of understanding the present and long-term consequences of injury both in a physical and an emotional context.

Throughout the summer, Dr. Gerding shared his experiences and manner of living with me. We spoke often about what it was like during medical school, clinical rotations, and residency, and how it was possible to be a surgeon and have a family at the same time. We also spoke about patients at the hospital, specifically their treatment and progress. We even discussed ethical issues such as when is a treatment prolonging death versus prolonging life.

While the discussions did not always have answers, they

were always rewarding and insightful. During the time we spent together I learned about becoming a doctor.

I shall always look up to Dr. Gerding for convincing me that medicine was definitely my calling. Prior to meeting him, I thought it was. After working with him, I knew it was.

Chapter 17

Blood Shooting Onto My Shirt

While I was a Chester Summer Scholar at Cleveland Metro General Hospital in the summer of 1986, Dr. Robert Gerding and I worked together to develop a model to test various drugs on rat burn shock mortality. I learned to anesthetize rats, to perform microsurgical cannulation (threading a very narrow tube into an even narrower blood vessel), and to suture. At first, cannulation seemed impossible. How could such a large tube be put into such a small vessel? With time it became possible and even facile.

While I first learned to cannulate, my mentor, Bruno Dodich, would assist me. He would do anything I requested during the procedure. I started the procedure by making an incision over the groin of a rat. I would dissect, find the femoral vessels, and then isolate the femoral vein. Once I had it isolated, I placed two untied sutures under the vein. I then tied the proximal suture (the one closest to the groin) and directed Bruno to gently pull upwards on the distal suture (farther from the groin). This would prevent bleeding from the next part of the procedure I had to perform. Using very delicate surgical scissors, known as Castroviejo scissors, I made a very small puncture into the femoral vein. The puncture had to be just large enough to insert the cannula, but not so large as to cut through the vein. I would then carefully thread the cannula into the vein until I reached the point of Bruno's suture. I then directed him to gently relax the tension as I continued threading the cannula into the vein. Finally, I tied his suture to secure the cannula in place.

One day, as I was about to request his assistance, he told me that he was not going to help anymore.

"But I will not be able to do it without your help," I said.

To this he replied, "I know you can do it."

Since there was no choice, I proceeded.

I started with the vein first. I isolated the femoral vein and tied a proximal suture and then placed another suture distally. This time, however, there was no one assisting me with the distal suture and I became nervous. After nearly an hour, with perspiration dripping down my face, I was ready to give up, but I did not. I persevered and finally succeeded. I designed a way to make a pair of hemostats the equivalent of a pair of hands. It took time to adjust, but I did. What a sense of accomplishment!

The artery, however, was still waiting, and it was going to be more difficult to cannulate than the vein. There was tremendous resistance due to the pressure in the artery. How would I be able to release the pressure on the distal suture without the flow of blood pushing the cannula out of the artery? And, if that happened, I would have only seconds to act, otherwise the rat would bleed to death.

On the first try, the cannula was forcefully pushed out of

the artery just as I had predicted. Blood shot out powerfully onto my shirt and the field quickly filled with blood. I knew I only had a few seconds to act. I did. I stopped the bleeding quickly, almost instinctively, by reapplying the pressure to the distal suture. Then I cleared the operating field. I tried again unsuccessfully. I tried for more than an hour, though it seemed like an eternity. I felt physically and emotionally drained.

Finally, my teacher, Bruno, who had once been my assistant, asked if I wanted help.

"No, not yours," I replied. "I'm not giving up yet."

I did not have many chances left. The rat was in hypovolemic shock from the blood loss and one or two more unsuccessful attempts would surely result in death. On the next try, I succeeded. I did it and without any help! Bruno was right. I *could* do it.

I am pretty sure about two hours into the procedure he changed his mind and *didn't* think I could do it, but I finally convinced him. In a matter of weeks I was doing the procedure in 15 minutes flat and that included the prep. I even began cannulating the femoral artery just to see if I could do it. This was a real challenge. The rats were between 200 and 250 grams (about 1/2 pound) and the femoral artery was the size of a very narrow wire. The procedure approached the limits of the unaided human eye, but somehow I was able to do it and it felt great.

Bruno, to this day, the lesson you taught me is one I shall never forget. Even when it seems beyond your capacity, don't give up!

Chapter 18

The Flight That Changed My Life

I attended Case Western Reserve University because I got a full tuition scholarship and was guaranteed a slot into their medical school. That guarantee was made to me upon my acceptance as a freshman in college (1984). After my first winter in Cleveland, I had serious doubts about remaining in Cleveland for another four years after college. Perhaps the most convincing moment came in January of 1985. That month the temperature never broke freezing and it snowed almost every day.

Upon returning from my junior year abroad in London, I had to start the process of applying to medical school. Even though I had the guaranteed slot at CWRU, my intent was to go somewhere else. Now it was as if I was just like any other premed student—I had to go through the formal process of applying unless I wanted to remain in Cleveland. I did not.

A very good friend of mine was a graduate student in chemistry at the time. His name was Dan Batzel. Dan encouraged me to apply to medical school at Stanford

University. Initially, this seemed like a ridiculous idea. Why would I go to California? I thought about it a little more and decided to call my high school friend, Terry Yen. He was attending Stanford University as an undergraduate at the time. When I spoke with him, he thought I should apply to both Stanford *and* UCSF. UCSF? I'd never even heard of UCSF. It was one of the University of California (UC) schools. It was the only UC School that had no undergraduates. UCSF had a medical school, dental school, pharmacy school, and nursing school. On the West Coast it was very well known. It turned out it was ranked one of the top 5 medical schools in the country and it was a state school.

At the time, I initially told my friend Dan there was no way I would apply in California. There was no possible way I would go there. Besides, I could barely afford more application fees. At the time, it cost around $50 to apply to medical school and I was applying to about 10 already. He encouraged me further. Given what Terry Yen said, I decided I'd apply to both Stanford and to UCSF. After doing so, I knew I'd still never go. There was absolutely no way I could afford to make a trip to California even if I was granted an interview at Stanford or UCSF.

In November of 1987 I was going home to New York for Thanksgiving. I took the train from the CWRU campus in Cleveland to the airport. On the way to the airport I felt certain that my flight home would be overbooked. It was Thanksgiving, and flights were always full and full flights at that time were often oversold. Sure enough, when I got to the airport, the flight was overbooked and they needed volunteers to take a later flight. I volunteered. In return for volunteering, I got a free round trip ticket anywhere in the United States.

Not long afterwards, Stanford contacted me and told me

they wanted to interview me for their medical school. Immediately I called UCSF and advised them that I had also applied to Stanford and that Stanford had granted me an interview. UCSF then decided to grant me an interview as well and they coordinated it to occur at the same time I was going to interview at Stanford.

Now that I had my free round-trip ticket, I decided to fly to California and interview, just as Dan had encouraged me to do all of those months ago. As soon as I saw UCSF, I knew I would accept an offer if they made me one. It was the 3rd or 4th top ranked medical school in the country at the time and in-state tuition in 1988 was $1,000 per year—**for medical school**! Out of state residents had to pay an additional $5,000, so my first year tuition would be $6,000. They made me an offer. I of course accepted.

Twelve months later I became a California resident. In 1989, tuition went up to $2,000. In 1990, it went to $3,000 and in 1991, the start of my fourth year of medical school, it went to $4,000. My *entire* tuition for four years of medical school was $15,000.

Had it not been for that oversold flight and getting voluntarily bumped, my entire life would have turned out differently.

Chapter 19

Strange on the Inside
or the Outside?

Six months or so after that free round-trip ticket got me to California I started medical school at UCSF. It was 1988. My experience two years earlier with burn and trauma surgeon Dr. Gerding made me think that I would be a surgeon. Once I started medical school it didn't take long to figure out that I would *not* be a surgeon. I think the top reason I decided against surgery was that I seemed to have nothing in common with my classmates who wanted to be surgeons.

At the end of my first year of medical school, another experience from my relatively recent past came back to me. In particular, my experience with Bruno Dodich, operating on rats. UCSF had a variety of opportunities for medical students to do research at the end of their first year of medical school. I decided to work with Dr. Ted Kurtz, a physician who worked in the department of laboratory medicine. He was young, bright, friendly and focused. I only had two months to do research that summer, so I needed to work in a lab that was focused, otherwise there was no chance I would accomplish anything meaningful in a short period of time. I knew I had an excellent opportunity with Dr. Kurtz. I was correct. Just like when I worked with Bruno, one of my jobs was to place cannulas into rats. Our study related to the inheritance of a specific gene associated with high blood pressure in rats. This investigation also raised the possibility that abnormalities of this gene, or a closely related gene, could be connected to increased blood pressure in one of the most common forms of elevated blood pressure in humans. It was a productive and excellent summer and resulted in a publication on our research.

Ted (Kurtz) and I got along famously. He was very amiable and I could relate to him like an older brother or uncle. At the start of the summer he told me I should be a dermatologist. Initially, I thought that was a ridiculous suggestion. Why would *anyone* want to be a dermatologist? He related that he had a good friend, Dr. Chuck Ellis, at the University of Michigan, who was a dermatologist. Ted said Dr. Ellis loved what he did and that dermatologists in general felt the same way. I wasn't really convinced, at least not yet.

My next dermatology exposure was with Dr. Howard Maibach. He led a series of weekly meetings with a small group of about 5 or 6 medical students and I was one of them. Dr. Maibach was not only a clinical dermatologist, he did a lot of basic science research relating to dermatology. I remember a few things about Dr. Maibach. He wore a bow-tie. He had an interesting voice. One day, he took my group of students to get coffee and pastries — he was both generous and kind.

Most professors would not do this sort of thing. I also remember his passion. Specifically, he said he *loved* what he did. He said that even at 3 a.m. in the morning he *loved* what he did. The sincerity of his statement stuck with me. And then I remembered what Ted Kurtz said about his friend Dr. Ellis. Perhaps there really was something to Ted's point about becoming a dermatologist.

As you go through medical school, and try to decide what type of doctor you want to be, it is apparent that liking the field matters, but equally important is liking the people who practice in that field. I think you have to see yourself as one of them and to do so you have to ask yourself if you like them. I liked Dr. Maibach and could see myself doing something that he liked doing. The genuineness of his passion was contagious.

As my second year of medical school continued, I thought ahead to my last two years, namely the ones where you do clinical rotations. Prior to starting my clinical rotations, I was favoring just two fields, dermatology and psychiatry. For whatever reason, it seemed that I either wanted to deal with things that were strange on the inside (psychiatry) or the outside (dermatology).

To this day, I am still not sure why I really considered psychiatry at all, but I did. As it turned out, my first clinical rotation was psychiatry. It was the start of my third year of medical school. Within a day or two of starting my psychiatry rotation I was convinced there was *no possible way* I would be a psychiatrist. I'm not sure this is relevant, but one of the few clinical rotations that I did not receive an honors grade in was psychiatry. Go figure!

After I completed my psychiatry rotation, I began doing some of my required clinical rotations, such as internal medicine, pediatrics, surgery, family medicine, Ob-gyn, and the like. I found a variety of fields interesting. For instance,

Ob/Gyn. I thought Ob/Gyn was very exciting and I liked the doctors in the field. But somehow there was no way I could see myself actually *being* an Ob/Gyn. Another field where I particularly liked the doctors was pediatrics. Pediatricians were very calm, easy going, and fun to work with. Well, I liked the *doctors*, but crying babies were not my cup of tea. I also liked the idea of emergency medicine, but thought there would be a high risk of burnout. As noted earlier, I didn't seem to fit the personality type of a surgeon, and I wasn't all that interested in internal medicine.

In the summer of my third year of medical school, I did my first dermatology rotation. By then, knowing it was the specialty I wanted to pursue, I began reading some basic textbooks of dermatology. I seemed to have the passion of learning dermatology in the same way that Dr. Maibach had practicing it. I was quickly able to assimilate the basic classification of dermatologic disorders. I also found that I had a good visual memory, so combining what I saw with what I read, I was learning quickly. In the time I was on that rotation I had a knowledge base that allowed me to respectably diagnosis the four or five most common diagnoses in most categories of dermatologic disease.

I expressed my desire to become a dermatologist while doing this rotation and I do not think it took long for the residents and attending physicians to realize my interest in dermatology and my growing knowledge base. The head of my rotation, a fairly well known dermatologist, Dr. Richard Odom, wrote in my review: "Excellent performance. He is interested in pursuing the specialty of dermatology. His dermatology knowledge is far beyond the average student." He also wrote, "Hopefully he will be allowed to rotate in dermatology again (i.e., inpatient service)."

If you wanted to follow the party line, and do things the politically correct way, you did your second rotation in inpatient dermatology. Personally, this idea never interested me. At the same time, I knew full well what Dr. Odom had written. It wasn't a subtle hint about the inpatient service. The clear message was, "If you want to do your dermatology residency at UCSF, *take* the inpatient dermatology rotation."

One day in my third year of medical school I was doing an internal medicine rotation and overheard the name Marcus Conant. I knew that name. Dr. Conant was one of the first doctors in the country to recognize that young, mostly gay men, were appearing with a very rare cancer, Kaposi's sarcoma. This cancer was usually seen in older men of Mediterranean descent and it was seen only rarely. In the early 1980s it was being seen more and more commonly—at an alarming rate. It was being seen in a pattern very different from the one seen in the older men. It was in fact soon recognized to be a manifestation of AIDS. Dr. Conant was known for being one of the first doctors in the country to recognize the presenting skin findings in patients with AIDS. He had also become a proponent for HIV research, community activity, and the like. He was such an important medical figure for AIDS that the book *And the Band Played On,* describing the HIV epidemic, included him. The book was written in 1987, just before I started medical school. It was adapted into an HBO movie in 1993 with Richard Jenkins playing Dr. Conant.

Presumably, by pure chance, I encountered a physician who worked with Dr. Conant while I was doing a rotation at a hospital that he worked at. Hearing his name and knowing his role in recognizing HIV, I seized on the opportunity. I asked his colleague to get me a meeting with Dr. Conant. She did.

I met Dr. Conant and told him I wanted to do a rotation with him for a month and publish something with him. I realized doing this was political death from the standpoint of the UCSF department of dermatology. Medical students who wanted to do dermatology residencies at UCSF *did* the inpatient rotation. The problem here was simple. I only had one elective month left for the duration of medical school. Inpatient rotation or Dr. Conant?

I chose Dr. Conant. Only once in a lifetime does an opportunity like working with such a physician come along. However, tears were shed about a year and half afterwards (more on that later).

I did my month with Dr. Conant. I got to spend time with him clinically, personally, and writing a paper about Kaposi's sarcoma. Dr. Conant was a genius of a clinician. Even when the rarest of things presented in his office, he was facile at diagnosing them. He had a great rapport with his patients. He was well respected. He was a community leader. He did research to try and make a difference in the AIDS epidemic. He stood up for policies to try and reduce the spread of AIDS. He had the same passion I witnessed in Dr. Maibach.

Dr. Conant retired relatively recently. He remained the same active figure, researcher, physician, humanitarian, and advocate throughout his career and I had the opportunity to spend a whole month working with him. *Wow!*

I dug out Dr. Conant's review of my time with him. He wrote: "Steve is perhaps the brightest and best organized student I have had the pleasure of working with in many years." Just thinking about passing up the opportunity to work with Dr. Conant versus working on the inpatient dermatology service makes me want to vomit.

Approximately one year after working with Dr. Conant I

was one of the authors on a review article about Kaposi's sarcoma. It covered just about everything there was to know about this cancer including its treatment. Treating Kaposi's sarcoma was one of the things that I reviewed in detail while working with Dr. Conant. I am forever thankful for the opportunity that Dr. Conant gave me and for my courage to tell the system to kiss my ass—take your inpatient service and shove it. Ok, that's not what I told them, it's what I thought.

The chance that the inpatient service would have helped me to become a better dermatologist, physician, or person was slim. Working with Dr. Conant forever impacted me as a physician and person. I do feel positive though that my decision to work with Dr. Conant cost me a residency position at UCSF.

I think Dr. Odom knew of my intent to work with Dr. Conant and thus intentionally put the statement about working on the inpatient service in my review. Am I bitter about this? I don't think bitter is the right word. I think I realized that life is short. Sometimes you take one opportunity which requires you to forego another. Working with a true leader and genius was my calling. There are 1,000,000 physicians in the United States. I would estimate there are less than 100 who have impacted our society in a way as important as Dr. Conant.

About a year and a half after working with Dr. Conant, while I was at UCLA doing my internship, the results of the dermatology match came in the mail. When I read the result, I cried. I was now going to have to do my residency (3 years) in Los Angeles. I had ranked UCSF as my top choice for dermatology residency and Harbor-UCLA as my second choice. I did not get my first choice.

It was Conant for life, or the inpatient service at UCSF for three more years in San Francisco. A life experience is more important, but I cried nonetheless. Fortunately, I didn't hate LA nearly as much as internship.

Thank you Marc. You touched thousands and thousands of lives in your career. Mine was one of them.

Chapter 20

My 30 Days of Addiction

In 1992, I got married, finished medical school, and started my medical internship at UCLA. I hated my internship. In the early 1990's, if you wanted to become a dermatologist, you had to apply for internship and dermatology residency separately. The process for applying was called "THE MATCH." Basically, graduating medical students applied to multiple programs and each program interviewed multiple candidates. Then applicants ranked the programs in order of their preference for acceptance. Likewise, programs created their own rank order list of applicants. All of the information was put into a computer and voila, this was "THE MATCH" and determined where you would do your training. Since you had to do an internship (one year) before dermatology residency (three years) you had to match in two separate processes.

In 1992, nearly every medical specialty had all of the matches occur on the same date. So, let's say you wanted to be a radiologist, you would apply for an internship (usually in internal medicine) and a separate radiology residency. On the day of the match, you found out both where you were going for internship and also where you would be going for residency.

Dermatology was one of the only fields that had what was known as a late match. So by the time I finished my 4th year of medical school in June, I found out the match results for my internship. However, the match for dermatology was delayed and did not occur until the fall of my internship year.

Why the difference for dermatology? Presumably, because dermatology is such a competitive field, residency programs decided that delaying the match gave them one more piece of information to decide who they would accept. So, unlike most fields where grades, standardized test scores, experiences, and letters of recommendation were enough, dermatology required one extra piece of information. Namely, where is this candidate going to do their internship?

The result of this was that almost all medical students who desired to become dermatologists had to attend very high powered and academic internships at big name medical centers if they wanted to be competitive candidates. This was one of many political parts of securing a coveted dermatology residency position. So I, like most of the other 300 or so people who would be accepted into dermatology residencies in the United States, went to places like UCLA for internship. Many hundreds more who applied to dermatology residencies did not get accepted into any dermatology program.

My intent, since my third year of medical school, was to be a dermatologist. If the match occurred simultaneously for internship and dermatology residency, I undoubtedly would have gone to an excellent community hospital. And while there, I would have seen the average things that got people hospitalized—like heart attacks, pneumonia, blood clots, and infections. Instead, playing the political game required to get into dermatology, I chose UCLA.

UCLA Medical Center was and still is a high-powered tertiary, referral based, complex medical center. They perform procedures and take care of patients that many medical centers would not be comfortable treating.

My first rotation, straight out of medical school, was oncology. My "call schedule" was every four nights. That meant that every 4th night for a month I would be up all night taking care of my patients, patients of the other interns rotating in oncology, and admitting new patients. The start of each "call day" began around 6 a.m., continued through the day, that night, the hours of the morning and all of the next day until around 6 p.m. It was a 36-hour shift, repeating itself every fourth day. Oncology, of course, was particularly difficult as many patients had terminal diseases. Others did not necessarily have terminal illnesses, but they often went through treatment that was hell. It was hard watching this and taking care of them.

Now also imagine yourself just coming out of medical school and having virtually *no* experience doing this and realizing that your care could literally *kill* a patient. At night, in particular, you had much less supervision than during the day.

At UCLA, there were two separate oncology related services. One was solid oncology. That service treated patients with cancers that are not related to the blood system such as lung cancer, colon cancer, breast cancer and the like. The other service was the bone marrow transplant service which generally took care of patients with leukemia or lymphoma.

My initial rotation was solid oncology, though every time I

was on call on the solid oncology service, I also had to cross cover the bone marrow transplant service's patients at night.

The bone marrow transplant service was one of the most overwhelming experiences I had as an intern. These patients required bone marrow transplants to either try to treat or cure their cancer. To accomplish a bone marrow transplant, you had to completely *destroy* a patient's bone marrow by using chemotherapy and radiation. Then, when they had no marrow left, you had to infuse bone marrow (sometimes their own that was treated, sometimes a relative's, sometimes a stranger's) and hope it would reconstitute the blood cells required to survive. These patients had a predicted statistical probability of surviving the transplant.

For instance, they could have an 80 or 90% chance of surviving the bone marrow transplant or a 10 or 20% chance of dying in a short period of time (often the first 100 days) after the transplant. Of course this treatment was almost always done because, without the bone marrow transplant, they faced a near certain death. The hope was that they would survive the transplant and also survive many more years afterward.

My first rotation, the solid oncology one, as noted, required me to cross cover the bone marrow transplant service every fourth night. So even though I wasn't caring for the patients on the bone marrow transplant service during the day, I was one of their key physicians between 6 p.m. and 6 a.m. the following morning. Another thing that the patients on the bone marrow transplant service had in common, in addition to facing possible death in 30 or 60 or 90 days, was that many of them were young. It was particularly difficult to see someone young go through this.

Medical school spent almost no time teaching you how to

deal with this. In a sense, medical school often *shielded* you from the extreme morbidity and mortality faced in my solid oncology and bone marrow transplant experiences. In fact, I took care of only a small number of patients with serious cancers while I was in medical school.

At UCLA, I had not one rotation in oncology, but two. My second rotation came a few months after my first. That one was the bone marrow transplant service. It too had a call schedule every fourth night (working from 6 a.m. one day until 6 p.m. the following day) and repeating every 4 days. Though I didn't comment much about the lack of sleep on my first oncology rotation, you might surmise that sleep was a five-letter word I didn't see much of at UCLA. I certainly didn't see it on the solid oncology or bone marrow transplant rotations.

If you put the strain of severe exhaustion on top of the extreme morbidity and mortality that I saw every day, you could see how overwhelmed you would feel coming out of medical school. Basically, you got virtually no sleep when you were on call, and out of each month rotation, you had only one day off. One day to attempt to recover from the physical and emotional exhaustion of 100+ hour work weeks taking care of horribly sick patients who were undergoing devastating treatments and sometimes died from the treatments. If this one day off per month was supposed to recharge your battery, it felt like the wall receptacle had a short in it.

Fortunately, I was not alone while on these rotations. Every rotation I was on had a supervising resident. They would always back you up and help you. Each resident had two interns to supervise. Basically, we interns had to round on every patient, get data on how they were doing, write orders, write admission and discharge notes, handle calls and questions, be the patient's doctor, interface with the families, deal with imminently life threatening emergencies, interface with fellows and attending physicians and try to keep our heads on straight during all of this.

The first thing I would do every day was see each patient who I was taking care of. This usually began around 6 a.m. and lasted an hour and a half or so. A little later, I'd meet with my other intern on my team and our resident. Around 8 a.m. the whole service would meet. There would be two teams, each with one resident and two interns, an oncology fellow and an oncology attending physician. The fellow and the attending physician made most of the key treatment decisions such as which drugs to administer and when to perform a transplant. They were basically the ultimate decision makers of therapy and intervention. The interns, including myself, were more data collection experts and the ones who took care of almost all of the other less serious decision making. We did a lot of the labor intensive and time consuming things. When we rounded with the fellows and attending physicians, we discussed how each patient had done in the past day and made decisions on their care for that day and going forward.

One patient, who I still remember fondly, was Mr. Kraft. Mr. Kraft was 39 years old (a decade younger than I am now while writing this book). He had CML, a form of leukemia that can go into a phase that can quickly be terminal. His best chance of cure was to have a bone marrow transplant. He went through all of the conditioning phases, including chemotherapy and radiation, and then Mr. Kraft received his transplant.

The transplant itself is a rather complicated thing. Let's assume you get a transplant from someone very unrelated to you genetically—your body will attack the transplant as foreign cells, the marrow won't successfully take up into your body, and you will die. Now let's assume the marrow is a perfect or near perfect match genetically. Your body won't recognize it as foreign, so that is good, but the marrow can in fact attack *your* body. The process goes like this. Your marrow with cancer is killed. The matched marrow is infused. It takes up residence in your body and survives and repopulates your body with white cells, red cells, and platelets. A short time later it *attacks* your body. This is called graft-versus-host-disease. This too can kill you. It killed Mr. Kraft.

I recall that Mr. Kraft was hospitalized on the private floor of UCLA. This floor had large, beautiful rooms, was very comfortable, and had amazing food. Seemingly, if you had to go through the extreme treatment required for a bone marrow transplant it only seemed fair that you should get to stay somewhere comfortable. While in that spacious room with food fit for a king, Mr. Kraft's bone marrow transplant started to attack his body. This process attacked his skin, his colon, and his liver. It resulted in a devastating rash, recalcitrant diarrhea, and worsening liver failure including progressive jaundice.

I recall that Mr. Kraft never had an appetite. One day his dinner consisted of monstrous sized shrimp and delectable, mouth watering vegetables. It looked better than entrees I had eaten at fancy restaurants. He asked if I wanted to eat it. I could not accept. No matter how little he could eat, even if I was bordering on starvation, I could not eat his food. It would never have seemed appropriate.

Mr. Kraft's father was always with his son. He was very supportive and I could see how it ate him up knowing what we all knew. Mr. Kraft was not going to survive. All the residents, fellows, and attending physicians did everything they could. They tried to get the graft to relent and stop attacking Mr. Kraft. It did not. I suspect we all had to accept our powerlessness. I hated it too.

That experience was one of the most difficult I faced in my year at UCLA. Later (I'm not sure how much), I termed the disease Graft-versus-Kraft. I'm not sure if this vague attempt at humor really helped at all. Ultimately, it's just one of the many stories of sheer human emotion and medical hardship that I as a physician faced along with my patients.

My other 10 months at UCLA were mostly no more of a picnic than what I described above. It is just a glimpse into why I said at the beginning of this chapter that I hated internship. When the end of December of 1992 came, I recall New Year's Eve. It was the worst New Year's Eve of my life. Two patients simultaneously coded (hearts stopped) while I was doing a rotation in the CCU (coronary care unit). One of those patients, Jimmy Nakamura, was awaiting a cardiac transplant. A matching heart had not yet become available. Jimmy coded and died that night.

The other patient who coded received every possible Hail Mary attempt to save his life. The attending physician came in at about 3 a.m. and was running (making decisions) the code. That patient survived. I do not remember his name. That night reminded me of taking care of Mr. Kraft. I and the other physicians were ultimately powerless in saving Jimmy Nakamura just like we were in saving Mr. Kraft. If only a matching heart had been available, but it wasn't.

About 3 weeks before that New Year's Eve I recognized something mathematical. I've always been a math whiz. Numbers fascinated me from the time I was in elementary school. The fascinating number here was 200. At the beginning of December of 1992 I did a calculation and knew when I had exactly 200 more days of internship left.

When the 200-day mark had crossed, I would come to work each day knowing the number of days left until I would be finished with my internship. I am thinking I cracked below the 200 mark sometime during my rotation on the bone marrow transplant unit. Some of my patients had less than 200 days to *live*. Now thinking back on this experience, I was counting my 200 days until *freedom*. As I said, that's how much I hated internship. Looking back on my year of internship, I can say it is perhaps the closest I ever came to thinking of suicide. An extra month of oncology or the CCU and I'm not sure if I would have taken my own life. I am glad to be alive to tell this and all the other stories in this book.

Each week that passed took my number lower and lower. 171 days until internship is over. 142 days until internship is over, and so on. It was around the end of May 1993, that the count finally fell to 30 days. It was at this time that my addiction began. Each day I came to work I recognized how close I was to being done with internship. It was as if I was on an illegal or controlled substance. I felt like I was high. I didn't know the name of the drug I was on, but it sure felt like I was on one. Every day I was a little happier than the last. 24 days to go. 19 days to go. It was like I was on amphetamines. I was flying high. I suspect in the final 10 days, it must have felt like I was shooting up again and again. I made it. I had survived. I finished what was undeniably the worst year of my life. I was 27 years old.

For years I had nightmares about those experiences. I dreamt that I had to repeat internship or another month on the CCU or the bone marrow transplant unit. Fortunately, each year that passed, I had fewer nightmares. I probably haven't had one for the last 5 or more. Writing this chapter is the closest I've come to having one in a long time. Sadly, while editing, I had this dream again.

THE END
(of one chapter of my life)

.

.

.

.

.

.

.

THE BEGINNING
(of another)

Chapter 21

Try Again. Again. Again. Again.

What Bruno Dodich taught me in 1986 has been a theme that has repeated itself multiple times in my life. Of course when he taught me the lesson that I was ready to cannulate a small vein or artery with no help it was because of his understanding of what my skills were and what they could be. It is sort of like riding a bike with training wheels and then taking them off. If you can ride with training wheels, the next progression would be to ride without them. Bruno knew just when to take the wheels off.

One of my passions in dermatology residency was taking photographs of interesting dermatologic diseases. In my first year of residency I made the decision to purchase a camera known as the Dental Eye Camera. It had a massive 100 mm macro lens. The lens was the better part of a foot long when not extended all the way. When it was extended, it was over a foot! Essentially the largest thing I could frame into a photo was the area between your waist and your neck, give or take.

On the other hand, I could photograph your palm and have it take up the entire photo, not to mention the clarity of the camera was so great, I could then submit your palm photograph to the FBI and they would have all the detail required to identify you. The hardest thing about deciding to purchase this camera was its cost. Back in 1993 when I bought it, the cost was right about $1000. That was a *lot* of money for a resident, but I never regretted buying it.

I did my dermatology residency at Harbor-UCLA Medical Center in Torrance, California. My program director (a saint in his own right), Dr. Arnold Gurevitch, provided the film (this was still several years before digital photography became popular) and covered developing costs. Since we used these photos for teaching purposes, they were developed into Kodachrome slides. Every photo I took was made into two slides, one for Dr. Gurevitch (Arnie) and one for me. By my third year of residency, I had accumulated almost 3000 photos. I had essentially become our residency program's photographer.

Sometime around my third year of residency I became aware that the *New England Journal of Medicine* had a section called Images in Clinical Medicine where they published a photo and brief description of some interesting medical entity. Simple, I now was on a mission: to get one of my photos published in the *New England Journal of Medicine*. The first photo I submitted was of a patient with scurvy. I diligently wrote a one-page summary and mailed it to the journal along with my photograph. A few weeks later I got a letter from the journal. They declined my submission. I was rejected. No big deal, since I had 2,999 more photos left.

Within a week, I wrote another summary, this time of a ritual known as cupping. This ritual was done by a South

Korean patient of mine for knee pain. Basically a cup is heated with an open flame. Then the cup is placed over the skin. As the air in the cup cools, it contracts, creating a vacuum, drawing the skin slightly inside. This mobilizes blood flow, which is thought to promote healing. My patient had a peculiar pattern of pigmented circles around a portion of his knee where this ritual had been carried out. I thought the photo was excellent so I submitted it. Once again, a few weeks later I received another letter from the journal. They declined my submission. I was rejected again. Again, no big deal, I had 2,998 more photos left.

This process continued over several months. I never lost hope and I fully intended that I would get published in the *New England Journal of Medicine*. It was on my eighth or ninth submission that I submitted photos and wrote up an interesting short description about a man who cut his hand on a fish tank while cleaning it. This resulted in an infection known as fish tank granuloma. It is a cousin of tuberculosis. A few weeks after I submitted this article, I received another letter from the *New England Journal of Medicine*. This time my letter was a letter of acceptance. My article, published along with my phenomenal mentor, Dr. Arnold Gurevitch, was published in 1997.

I have another goal photographically and that is to publish a photograph in *National Geographic*. So far I have a lot more rejections than the *New England Journal of Medicine*, but I am not giving up on my goal. Perhaps I will have something to report back in my second book!

Part III

*Scrotal Surgery, Sterility, Paying For Sex
And More Observations*

Chapter 22

Books by Hugh Sless

...Required reading for Medical I/T professionals...

Almost every aspect of medical practice is now dominated by information technology (I/T) and it is completely unreliable. This includes messaging, scheduling, billing, prescriptions, dictation, connecting to the internet, and of course medical records. I'm sure I drove that point home earlier in *The Book of Excuses, Part II*.

The only way to combat this inefficiency and prevent myself from checking into the nearest looney bin is to crack jokes about it daily. Sadly, the I/T department just doesn't get my humor.

Undoubtedly, most required reading for medical I/T professionals, is written by the author Hugh Sless, whose numerous titles are published by a Russian conglomerate, Vasteov Paper.

Some of Hugh Sless's books that are required reading for medical I/T professionals are:

1. *Driving on 7 Out of 8 Cylinders*

2. *0-60 in 6.2 Seconds (+ 3 Days)*

3. *Why Crash Later If You Can Crash Now?*

4. *Make More Mistakes Get Paid More*

5. *How I Get Paid Even Though I'm Useless at My Job*

6. *Estimated Time for Accomplishment Unknown*

7. *Computer Crashed? Have you Tried Turning It Off and On Again?*

8. *I/T Dating Lessons: Have You Tried Turning it Off and On Again?*

9. *Upgrade Schmupgrade*

10. *Over-Promise and Under-Deliver*

* * *

Where I work is the NASCAR capital of the country. Strangely enough, one time I saw a help wanted ad for NASCAR. It read:

Wanted, sheet metal worker for NASCAR race team.
Must be highly experienced in working with crashes.
Desire 10 years or more experience working in I/T.

* * *

One Friday we got an email that the entire system was going down Friday night to do an upgrade. Our electronic medical record company, whose name I cannot share, assured us that everything would go just fine with the upgrade. Coincidentally, the top 20 executives of the company retired earlier that day and told us, "Don't call us, we'll call you."

One day I received a call from the I/T department wanting to know if I said that I/T sucked. I told them that was not what I said. Well, what I actually said was, "I/T sucks more than a Dyson/Hoover/Electrolux/Oreck hybrid vacuum cleaner on electrical steroids and crack cocaine." Fortunately, my I/T Department has a guarantee. The I/T Department printed this guarantee and sent it to all the offices of our group. Here's the guarantee:

Your computers are guaranteed to work 24/7*

* Except when you are at work

* Except when you need to use them

* Monday, Tuesday, Wednesday, Thursday, Friday and select weekends excluded

* Except when the patient does not remember what you treated them for and what you prescribed for them

---

The I/T department was coming to my office to do some repairs. I got a call that the department was in the I/T van and they were running late. The wireless connection to their GPS crashed and they couldn't find my office. They did not know where they were, OR, where I was.

Fortunately, my telephone system has a variety of helpful prompts. One prompt says, for directions, press 11. The I/T department still couldn't find my office.

They said their phone only had the numbers one through nine.

Chapter 23

HELGA AND OLGA

As a physician, one of the most annoying things is no-shows. What I am referring to here is patients who have an appointment and don't come to it. I believe this problem is rampant across all medical fields. In my estimation, even under the best of circumstances, I would say that approximately 10% of patients do not show up to their appointment.

To combat this problem, in my practice, EVERY patient is called prior to their visit with a reminder call. There were years that I had automated computer programs make these calls, but for most of my career it has been by one or more of my staff members. For certain patients, namely those with longer appointments or procedure visits, we make two reminder calls. Usually we do this two days before your visit and again one day before your visit. If we do not get a hold of you on either of those two days, we cancel your visit and we let you know we did this because you were unable to confirm. Note, we also advise you of this at the time we schedule one of those visits for longer appointments and procedures.

So why is it so annoying when someone does not come to their visit? There are many reasons. My staff and I have already prepared for your visit by checking your prior records, setting up surgical trays, arranging for medications to be available, prepared your chart notes, and like anything else we have a business to run. If you gave us a phone call telling us you needed to cancel or couldn't make it, and you gave us some advanced notice, (24 hours is what we request) we could easily fill your slot. Thus, when you don't show, someone else has to wait longer to be seen. And while many people think that physicians are grossly overpaid, the fact is that reimbursements have been dropping quickly and costs have been rising equally quickly. Thus, patients who don't show up to their visit cost resources and hurt our practice.

Some patients of course have good reasons for not showing up. They were in a car wreck, they have the flu, a family emergency came up, etc. Many of those patients *still* call and let us know. But we understand when they cannot. A large percent, however, simply "forgot" their appointment. Now if you just had a regular follow up visit say for eczema, this might not be such a big deal. But when you are scheduled for an hour-long surgical procedure, it is a huge deal. That's the reason we make *two* reminder calls for this type of visit and urge you of the necessity to give us at least 24 hours if you can't make it to your visit.

One day we called a patient, who we will call Johnson. I sure hope a lot of Johnsons aren't reading this book, because it is my number one name to use in a negative light, unless you work for I/T. In that case, *whatever* your name, I use it in a negative light. For those Johnsons reading, feel free to substitute the name *Smith*. Back to Johnson. So Johnson was scheduled for an hour-long surgery the next day. We had confirmed his visit and confirmed it again the day before. He stated he knew the time and would be there.

The next day comes and what happens? **Johnson is a NO-SHOW!** We call him up during his visit slot and he says, "I forgot." You forgot? You forget to get bread at the supermarket when your wife asks you to get milk and bread. How does someone forget they have an appointment for a surgery, especially after we called you twice and you confirmed? To make matters worse, instead of exhibiting an *ounce* of contrition, he was totally nonchalant about the matter. To him, it was no big deal. It happens. This pissed me off to no end.

Within 24 hours, I had created the following scenario. Johnson called back a few weeks later to reschedule and I answered the phone.

> **JOHNSON:** "I'd like to schedule a 60 minute surgery appointment to cut something off."

> **ME:** "Johnnnnson, Johnnnnson, Johnnnnson..... Say...weren't you the patient who missed their surgery visit a few weeks ago? The *sixty-minute* surgery slot that we had set aside for you? The one we confirmed the day before and you said you were coming to? You, ah, forgot, is that right?"

> **JOHNSON:** "Yeah, I need to reschedule it now."

> **ME:** "Johnson, I'm trying to remember what we had you scheduled for. You, ah, had a cyst I think......Yeah, a cyst........You had a cyst on your scrotum...........Yeah, a cyst on your *scrotum*, right?"

JOHNSON: "Yeah. It's been growing and is sore."

ME: "No problem Johnson. We'll schedule you for tomorrow. I'll have my two nurses assisting me with the procedure, HELGA and OLGA. They are the best. (static on the line........) I should let you know though, that HELGA has a slight resting tremor. She will be doing your numbing. She likes to drink double espressos for breakfast. She usually has 3 or 4. Why don't we schedule you first thing in the morning, just after she finishes breakfast? (static on the line)....Usually when she's numbing, she only has to enter the skin three or four times due to her tremor. But don't worry, she's really a very nice nurse and it shouldn't hurt TOO much." (static......)

JOHNSON: "Hey, doc, my cell phone reception was a little touchy there. You said your nurses Helga and Olga will be assisting you and you could schedule me first thing in the morning--*great!*"

ME: (static.......) "And during the actual surgery, OLGA will be assisting me. She is also a great nurse. She does have a slight hearing impairment." (static....)

JOHNSON: "Doc, speak up a little, my cell phone cut out."

ME: "Her hearing impairment acted up just a touch when we did our last scrotal cyst. She might have had an ear infection as well at that time. I was just finishing up another guy's surgery for his scrotal cyst. There was almost a little mishap during the surgery. It's a good thing I yelled loud at OLGA."

JOHNSON: "Doc, my cell phone signal is a little poor. Could you speak up?"

ME: "I still remember what I yelled. "OLGA, I said cut the **stitch** off, not the **dick** off!!!!"

JOHNSON: (static......) "You said you won't have to cut the stitches off. Great doc! Set me up."

ME: "Mr. Johnson, please hold on a minute, and I'll have one of our receptionists put you on the schedule. Oh, and it was *so* nice that you called back to reschedule. I was hoping that you would."

Fortunately, the number of surgery no-shows is pretty low. The number of "I forgot" patients though is *not* low. Out of my 100,000 separate patient encounters in nearly 20 years of being a dermatologist, I would estimate I have had at least 10,000 (that is not a typo) people not show up to their visit. So please do me a favor, be sure that you tell at least 10 of your friends how great a book this is so they can buy one too.

"OLGA! OLGA! Are you sure you wrapped Johnson's bandage tight enough? And be sure to use the *extra* sticky tape!"

Chapter 24

You'll Never Believe This

Practicing in medicine for just shy of 20 years has allowed me to have a lot of conversations with patients. Sometimes they are *very* interesting. I've taken a little poetic license on some.

ME: "Can I take a look in your mouth?"

PATIENT: "My mouth?"

ME: "Can I check your back?"

PATIENT: "My back?"

ME: "Are you a parrot?"

PATIENT: "A parrot?"

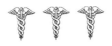

ME: "Yes, You have a spot on your arm. It's under your finger.............................. Well if you'll MOOOOOOVVVVVVEEEEEEE your finger OFF of the spot, maybe I can see it."

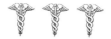

ME: "Can I check your abdomen?" (patient is sitting up on the exam table and I am sitting down on a stool in front of them).

PATIENT: (Lies back and pulls up their gown)

ME: "Simon did not say lie back and pull up your gown. I can see your abdomen with you sitting up, otherwise if "YOU" lie down, now *I'll* have to stand up to see your abdomen."

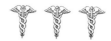

ME: "Can I check the spot on your arm?......Your leg?........Your butt?.........Your head? I am still trying to find the spot on your arm, but you just pointed to your leg, your butt and your head before I could take a look at your arm. Did you forget to take your ADD medication today?"

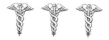

ME: "You had a spot a month ago and it fell off. What do I think it was? A scab. Next question."

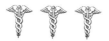

ME: "You see bugs on your skin. I recommend you use bug spray."

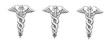

ME: "You think there are bugs IN your skin. Let me check. Yes, my colleague has an opening on their schedule next week to take a look."

As an interesting aside, there was the time I had to cut out two botflies that were embedded in a patient's skin and they in fact did tell me, "I have botflies in my skin."

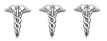

ME: "Do I think you are crazy? Are you sure you want my answer?"

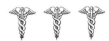

PATIENT: "That didn't hurt a bit."

ME: "We haven't done anything yet."

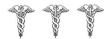

ME: "Does this hurt when I touch you?"

PATIENT: "Yes!"

ME: "It does? I haven't touched you yet!"

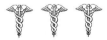

PATIENT: "I think I have bedbugs."

ME: "In that case I suggest you sleep on the couch"

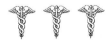

ME: "Hello Mr. S. You have a spot on your face."

Mr. S: "A spot? My face?"

ME: "Yes, you have a spot on your face?"

Mr. S: "What spot?"

ME: "The one on your face. It says *here on your note* that you have a spot on your face."

Mr. S: "A place."

ME: "Oh, you have a *PLACE* on your face. Fine. Let's take a look at the place."

Mr. S: "My place? Yeah, we're remodeling the kitchen. You want me to go back to my place?"

ME: "NO. I'm referring to the spot on your face. I mean the *place* on your face."

Mr. S: "Oh, *that* place..........It went away two weeks ago."

ME: "Excellent. Take this sheet up front to check out."

REALLY

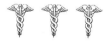

ME: "Yes, you have a spot on your arm?"

PATIENT: "My arm? No, it's ah, um, on my ah, penis."

ME: "But it says here on your sheet that you have a spot on your *arm*."

PATIENT: "I just told the nurse that. It's actually

on my penis."

ME: "In that case, I'll send the nurse in to take a look first."

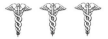

NEXT PATIENT..........

ME: "Yes, you have a spot on your arm. Let's take a look at your penis."

PATIENT: "My **PENIS**?"

ME: "Yeah, the last guy who said he had a spot on his arm said he told the nurse that because he didn't want to tell the nurse that the spot was on his penis."

PATIENT: "But I don't have a spot on my penis."

ME: "Oh, sorry. Let's take a look at your arm."

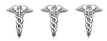

NEXT PATIENT..........

ME: "Let's take a look at your arm."

PATIENT: "Yeah doc, I got a spot on my arm, here."

ME: "That spot is a freckle, it's benign."

PATIENT: "I also got a rash on my feet."

ME: "Let's have a look. That's a fungus. I'll write a cream for you to use twice a day and it'll fix it up for you."

PATIENT: "I've also been losing my hair."

ME: "Yes, this is male pattern baldness. I recommend Rogaine. It's over the counter."

PATIENT: "I've also been having a rash on my hands for a few weeks."

ME: "That's eczema, here try this sample a couple of times a day."

PATIENT: "I've also got this mole that's changing colors."

ME: "That spot needs a biopsy, let's take care of it right now."

PATIENT: "Thanks for looking at my freckle, my athlete's foot, my hair loss, that rash on my hands and taking off that mole that's been changing colors, but Doc, none of those are the reason I'm here today though."

ME: "They aren't? You mean the *five* things we just took care of are *NOT* why you are here? Why are you here?"

PATIENT: "I've got a spot on my penis."

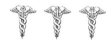

NEXT PATIENT..........

ME: "Boy, you'll never believe this! The guy I just saw had a spot on his penis. I mean, his **PENIS**. Can you believe some guy comes to see me with a spot on his **PENIS? HIS PENIS!** So how can I help you today?"

PATIENT: "I just got a call from work, can I

reschedule this visit?"

ME: "**YES!**"

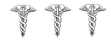

NEXT PATIENT.........

ME: "Yes, you have a spot where?"

PATIENT: "On my ass."

ME: "I'm sorry I didn't hear you. You have a spot where?"

PATIENT: "It's on my ass."

ME: "I'm really sorry, I still didn't hear you. Where?"

PATIENT: "On my ass."

ME: "Did you just say you have a spot on YOUR ASS? I'll send the nurse right in to take a look at it."

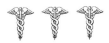

NEXT PATIENT.........

ME: "It says here you have a spot on your penis."

PATIENT: "Yes, I do."

ME: "My nurse will be right in to give you the name of one of my colleagues. He just moved here from Russia. His name is Dr. Tchopitov."

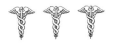

NEXT PATIENT..........

PATIENT: "Is this going to hurt?"

ME: "Me or **YOU?**"

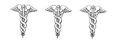

NEXT PATIENT..........

ME: "Mr. Johnson, hello, it's Dr. Wolfe. I'm calling to see how you are doing. How's that spot we froze on your penis doing?"

PATIENT: "It fell off."

ME: "The spot, or your penis?"

SCENARIOS I WISH WOULD HAPPEN BUT DON'T

"Mr. Johnson your insurance does not cover ANY of this evaluation. We charge the same way that lawyers do, by the minute. My fee is $450 per hour. That equals $7.50 per minute.

And yes, you have 12 problems you'd like addressed today.

Let's take it REAL slow.

Let's proceed.

Oh, and by the way, we run your credit card first for $5,000. We call that a "retainer," just like attorneys have."

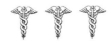

 "Mr. Johnson........

Your deductible is $5,000.

Today's visit will be $4900.

Wait........just a moment.

I think I hit the wrong button on the calculator.

Yes. I did.

Today's visit is $4990.

How would you like to pay?"

Steven F. Wolfe, MD

DR. WOLFE'S VISION TEST
(at least on some days)

IMVACKO

IMMOWRON

IMPAININASS

IMWEAKESTLINK

IGOTDARUNS

WHEREISDATOILET!

Fuhgettaboudit!

SOME DAYS FEEL LIKE THIS

ME: "Hello. May I speak to Mr. Wang?"

YOU: "Wang?"

ME: "Yes, Wang."

YOU: "Mr. Wang?"

ME: "Yes, Mr. Wang."

YOU: "Sorry, Mr. Wang stepped out."

ME: "Oh, in that case, can I speak to Mr. Wing?"

YOU: "Wing?"

ME: "Yes, Mr. Wing."

YOU: "Oh, Mr. Wing was outside all afternoon mowing the grass."

ME: "Outside?"

YOU: "Yes, outside."

ME: "It was really hot outside wasn't it?"

YOU: "Yes, really hot."

ME: "Is Mr. Wing OK?"

YOU: "No. Mr. Wing is hot. **HOT WING!**"

ME: "What about Mr. Wong?"

YOU: "I'm sorry, I think you have the WONG number. Only Mr. Wang and Mr. Wing work here."

ME: "What? I have the WONG number?"

YOU: "Can I put you on hold for a moment? The other line is winging."

ME: "I thought you said the phone WANG, am I WONG?"

YOU: "Who's on first."

ME: "That's right and what's on second."

Chapter 25

An AMAZING Cure For Sterility

It wasn't until I was in practice for 8 years that I finally got my own office. Prior to that, I worked in offices that were pretty plain Jane. You know the type. Wallpaper in boring patterns. Beige paint. Sterile chairs. Exam rooms that have diagrams of the intestinal tract or the lung. Exam tables that are an ugly green color. These are exactly the type of offices that I've been to when I have been a patient too.

Before I got my own office, I tried to exert a little bit of my own style into the offices that I had little control over. I put up some art, admittedly nothing stellar, but something more interesting than a flower. For a period of about 3 years, I would take cool stuffed animals, attach a string to them, and hang them from the commercial drop down grid ceiling. When I took care of younger children, I would let them pick their stuffed animal, then I pulled it down from the ceiling and gave the stuffed animal to them. And I virtually always gave out Dum Dums lollipops. I found these little things were unexpected, lightened the mood, and made people relaxed.

When I started the construction process of my current office it was imperative, at least to me, to do something way out of the ordinary. After all, I had waited 8 years to have my own office. My goal was to use a different paint color in every exam room. Likewise, I wanted it to contrast so that when you looked out of one room, down a hallway, into another, you could see multiple colors simultaneously. I had some excellent help in the design phase from a designer named Kay Kirby. Together, we chose the colors. Prior to the actual construction, I changed a few to make them even brighter.

I still remember when the painters cut in the borders around the door frames. This resulted in a relatively small strip of color around a white door frame. Even at that stage it looked amazing. Then, over a period of a few days, all of the color was in. At first, even for me, I thought it was too much. The lime green was *so* intense. The purples were great. The pink in my procedure room was soft and appealing. The yellow in the break room was bright and cheery. Over the years, what was too intense became too dull, and I had to change at least a room or two every 2-3 years.

One year, I decided to have a black and white cow pattern painted in the reception area. Before that, the area had been painted a soft peach color. To do the project, we had to take everything off of the walls. Then, my painter had to paint everything white and let it dry for a few days. I remember how sterile it looked. In fact, it was so depressing to me that I could tell the noticeable change in my mood as soon as I got to work. I could barely take it. The absence of art and colors was so dramatic that I didn't know how anyone could work that way. It was this stark *absence* of what I had been used to in my office that produced the amazing cure to this sterility.

Pure and simple, it was art, color, and design.

When the painters came back to paint the black to actually make the black and white cow pattern that I wanted, it was amazing and uplifting. The contrast to the sterility for those few days, and then that brightness, was very intense. My mojo was back.

Each time I have made a design change in the office it is immediately noticed and commented on by dozens of people within hours if not days. Now my office has a leopard pattern in my own back office, a Holstein cow pattern in the reception area, textured cobalt blue with sparkle contrasted with bright orange and bright lime green in the waiting room, pink with blue and black accents in one procedure room, purple with green accents in another procedure room, and brightness throughout. My art collection includes equally bright pieces, metal sculptures, three-dimensional pieces, and pieces from my travels. It also includes a large variety of photographs I have taken. I try to add pieces at least every 6-12 months.

When I first opened my office in 2004, we were closed on Wednesdays. I thought that we should rent out our space to a psychiatric practice on that day. I was convinced that we could run a depression clinic and have patients just sit in our exam rooms without any other treatment or intervention and that their mood would be better after leaving our office.

I always remembered the movie *Patch Adams* with Robin Williams and felt this was one of my ways to do something beyond the actual medical or surgical interventions I performed. I am still convinced that the *environment* in which you provide or receive your care can have as great an impact on your care as the actual medical care you receive. Likewise, each time we paint another area of the office and have to take everything down from the walls, I feel the change of my mood immediately to a much more somber one. And, upon completion of the project, the new brightness or contrast makes things even happier than they were before.

I truly don't know how I would practice in the absence of art, photography, and bright happy colors.

Chapter 26

Paying For Sex

I don't like lawyers. What does this chapter have to do with them? With the title "Paying For Sex," you would hope or think it would have a lot to do with them. In reality, this chapter has almost nothing to do with lawyers. This chapter is about the pharmaceutical industry. Well, there actually is one similarity that lawyers and the pharmaceutical industry have in common—I don't like either of them.

For the most part, the reps who have called on me during my career have pretty much used the same tactics. In fact, they could probably all swap each other's jobs and it wouldn't make much of a difference. In one way or another, they are all peddlers of products and are following a protocol from their company. Each company has the same protocol—sell our drug and make us money!

There are so many slimy tactics, it is despicable. One of the most common of course is to give doctors samples.

"Here doctor, have some free samples that you can give to

your patient then you can write our overpriced drug and skyrocket the cost of treating people. You see we have this new acne cream and it really is better than the old stuff. Oh, that old stuff? That has gone generic and it stinks. You see it was only available for 17 years as a brand when nothing else was available and it worked great. But now that it is a generic, and cheaper, it is horrible. Here, take some samples of my *unbelievably expensive* new medication and be sure to write lots of scripts for your patients."

What they don't tell you is that the drug costs 10 times as much as an acceptable generic.

"This acne cream (which costs $400 a tube) is great. It's well tolerated and effective. Oh, and our company never wants us to tell you that it costs $400 a tube. But if you ask us the price, we'll deflect your question immediately. Why our drug is *free*. See, here, we have a copay card. It will pay the $50 that the patient would otherwise have to spend. Give them the card and the drug is *free*."

"*Free? Really?* How much does the insurance company pay for it?"

"Well, uh, that price, it's negotiated. It's uh, not fixed. It depends on the company."

"I see. How much does United HealthCare pay for it?"

"Sorry doctor, I don't have that information available."

"How much does it cost for a patient with *no* insurance?"

They then look at you like you asked the most taboo question possible.

"Let's cut the crap. Tell me how much the drug costs or you'll never see it prescribed from me."

"Um. It's $400 a tube."

"$400 a tube, for an acne cream? Do I look like I was born yesterday?"

I mean I do, because I've been injecting an overpriced toxin into my own forehead for the last decade and I have almost no wrinkles. Oops, that was a digression.

So, back to one of those new acne medications. One came out that was a gel. It had the highest reduction of pimples of any medicine that had ever been studied. The efficacy was amazing when compared to the old standby, a drug that had the letter "A" in it for acne. Of course that "A" drug had now been available as a generic for a while. This new "highly" efficacious gel would literally tear your face off. If I gave it to a patient it was a guarantee that I'd have a call the next day that their face was red and felt like it was burned.

"Oh, your face is red and feels like it was burned (which it was)? Don't worry about it. This is the most efficacious drug out there."

So basically, if I wanted to USE this drug for a patient, this acne gel, I'd have to have a 15-minute discussion in great detail on how to use it and not burn your face off. You call this a breakthrough? I call it a ripoff!

Then there's the old swaparoo. Our old drug, which was great, has now gone generic. What did their company do? Let's say they had a 1% cream and it went generic. The rep would come to my office and tell me they had a new branded 1.1% cream.

"It is *way* better than the old 1% cream."

"How much does it cost?"

"It's *free*. Here's the copay card, doctor."

This copay card baloney is a pile of crap. It's a way to get an expensive drug to a patient and have the patient pay nothing or very little. It's also a way to avoid discussing the cost to _society_. I don't care what the patient pays, I care about what the cost to society is. I explain to every patient that it doesn't matter if I give you a drug that costs you nothing out of pocket. If your insurance has to pay $300 for it each month, it costs $3600 a year. And how do you think your company decides how much to raise your premiums next year? It is based on utilization (for example of $300 a month acne products).

"Doctor, I've got this great branded acne pill. It's the number one prescribed branded acne pill in the United States."

If cocaine is the number one abused illicit substance in the United States, does it mean I use it? You mean you've suckered my colleagues into writing it and you think you can do the same with me?

"OK. How much is this branded antibiotic to treat acne?"

"It's *free,* here's a copay card."

"Let's cut the crap. How much for a self pay patient?"

"Oh, we have a special offer for patients who are self pay and don't have insurance."

"OK, how much for someone with Medicare?"

You see, Medicare insurance is virtually always *excluded* from copay cards. Pharmaceutical companies can only thrive on things administered to Medicare patients *in* the office (like infusible drugs or medications applied in the office).

Back to the Medicare patient.

"My patient is disabled, 25 years old, and has Medicare. How much is the acne pill?"

"$900 a month."

"You freaking mean to tell me that it's $30 a pill to treat acne? **GET OUT OF MY OFFICE!"**

You see the sales talk is always like this.

"Doctor, I've got this new drug (it's the same as the old ones, but my company makes me tell you it's new). It is fantastic. Let's not talk about side effects though, I don't want to hurt my sales."

"What about the black box?"

"Oh, that black box (known as a warning on the package insert—things like you could die taking the drug, or patients have killed themselves while taking the drug, or the drug causes cancer, or might perforate your intestine), let's not talk about that. Here's a red box. It's some chocolates I brought for the office. Who wants to talk about black boxes (warnings) when we can talk about red boxes of dark chocolates."

Sadly, most doctors do see pharmaceutical reps, take samples, and use copay cards. I do not.

When I think about medications, I am always thinking about *value*. "What *value* does this drug offer? *Is* it a value? I see, you have a drug to treat rosacea. A pill. It's $483 a month to treat rosacea but it doesn't cure rosacea. My patient will have to stay on it indefinitely. You mean society will have to spend $6,000 a year to control rosacea, something that won't kill my patient, yet I can prescribe them a generic cholesterol pill for under $100 a month. A pill to treat something that *can* kill them? Let me see if I've got this right. I do. **Get out of my office!**"

Of course I have medicines to treat rosacea for a fraction of the cost, but the pharmaceutical rep and company don't want me to think about those *cost effective* ideas.

The number of drugs whose costs are rapidly skyrocketing continues to go up. But wait, we can now treat diseases we once couldn't. We can *cure* hepatitis C. It only takes 12 weeks to do it. The cost of treatment is $94,500. That's $1125 per pill. *Wow!*

Of course that's nothing compared to the most expensive medication in the world. It treats a rare disorder called paroxysmal nocturnal hemoglobinuria. It better be expensive if it treats something I can barely spell and you can barely pronounce. How expensive? Only $409,500 per year. Let me spell that out in case you think I typed it wrong. Four hundred nine thousand five hundred dollars a year!

In 2014, the top 25 drugs had revenues of $145 billion. The lowest selling one sold $2.7 billion. Sadly, for the company, this arthritis pill will lose its patent soon. Please get me a box of tissues, I'm about to cry.

The top selling drug is used in dermatology (amongst other things). I just went online to check its cost. Why it's only $3265 for a box that contains two injections, enough for 4 weeks. That's $42,445 for a year's use. It's no wonder this company keeps trying to get into my office. Of course when they used to come to my office (until I stopped letting them in) they would tell me why it was better than the competitor (the 5th best selling drug in the world, 2014 sales of $8.54 billion).

"But what about the part of the package that talks about the drug causing infections which can sometimes be fatal, and the risk of it causing cancer?"

"Let's talk about that the next time we come to see you doctor. Cost? What cost? Here's a 1-800 phone number. Call it and your patient will get the medication for *free!* We'll be glad to pay their portion for them, as long as their insurance company will fork out $35,000 or $40,000 for a year's worth. Oh, and that visit that I'll pay you to discuss the black box warnings? Let's put that off a couple of months. I was the top sales rep in my district and my husband and I just got a 2 week all-expenses-paid vacation to Hawaii from my company. Boy, my company is great to me! All I had to do was push a few million dollars of this drug to doctors like you."

Do you like government regulations? Is that a question even worth asking? For the most part, they create havoc in my professional life, making me be a bean counter and asking stupid questions like, "What's your first language?"

But you would think that with all the regulations we have from the government and insurance companies that we might be able to have some regulations that make sense and SAVE money. **Do you know that Medicare is NOT allowed to negotiate prices for drugs**? Perhaps you should re-read that sentence again. By law, Medicare has to pay exactly what the drug companies charge for any drug. Perhaps that's why one drug that I use to treat precancers of the skin has gone from $110 per dose to $300 per dose. I wonder if the company that sells this drug knew that Medicare cannot negotiate prices? And boy, this ObamaCare sure is great for pharmaceutical companies by creating a larger base of people to use expensive and often overpriced drugs.

Why is it that other countries have price caps on drugs and can negotiate based on therapeutic benefit?

Here, in the United States, I've got to listen to some tennis guy from Douglaston, New York whining about toenail fungus on TV. So ask your doctor about toenail fungus.

"I'm your doctor. Go ahead ask me!"

That drug—it costs $565 for a 4 ml bottle (about 1/7 of an ounce), has to be used for 48 weeks, will take 12 bottles to treat a *couple* of nails, and cost society about $6,500.

What about the cure rate? In the two studies done by the company, the 'complete cure' rate was 15.2% in one study and 17.8% in another. What if all of your nails were involved? Every day it would take two drops for each big toe nail, one drop for each of your other toenails and a bottle would last about a week. It would cost about $20,000 for one 48-week course of treatment.

When this drug was presented during a dermatology conference that I attended in early 2015, I asked the doctor giving the presentation about its cost. Actually, I threw a jab at him since I knew it cost $565 for a 4-week supply and needed 12 bottles for the treatment. Of course this was one of the doctors who did the study and was being paid by the company (probably dearly). He told me that it wasn't $565. He gave me the same crap the reps do. Well, the price is negotiated with each insurance company. Nobody pays the list price. There's copay cards. Yeah buddy, and you are as full of shit as the reps and the companies that make these drugs.

At the conference I let the course director know that I thought there should be *no* drug reps at our conference. He said that the cost of the conference would be prohibitive if we didn't have pharmaceutical funding.

Really? Let's look at the cost of the conference and see. Would you be willing to share those numbers with me?

Ah, well, um, *no*. The company that puts on the CME (continuing medical education) conference wouldn't let me share that with you. And besides, we get free breakfast and coffee with the pharmaceutical support. In fact, the course director said the price of coffee alone was like $15 a cup.

Really? I just bought some coffee at the hotel restaurant near my room. It was $2.

The numbers are simple. The conference costs about $500 for registration. There were roughly 350 attendees. With no pharmaceutical support, the registration would likely be $1000. Of course the director of the conference didn't want to divulge any information. Most course directors partake in thousands if not tens of thousands of dollars in profit for putting on these types of conferences. I wonder if he'll like the t-shirt I'm going to wear to his conference in 2016. The one with the cover of this book. Go ahead, ask me what my book is about!

Sadly, in my field, almost all conferences have pharmaceutical support. Not so in many primary care conferences. I've attended several primary care conferences put on by two respected companies. They have *no* pharmaceutical support. The information is unbiased. I don't think it is unbiased at my dermatology conferences. Shame on my conferences for being in bed with the pharmaceutical industry.

And why does a stomach acid medicine, a little colored pill, cost about $250 a month in the United States when it costs $60 in Switzerland and $23 in the Netherlands? And how come a cancer drug that cost $28,000 a year in 2001 cost $92,000 in 2012 for the exact same drug?

The number of drugs costing over $100,000 per year tripled from 2013 to 2014! In 2014, more than 500,000 people in the United States had annual drug costs that exceeded $50,000. Likewise, in 2014, the expenditure on cancer drugs in the US topped $100 billion. As noted earlier, we can cure hepatitis C at a cost of approximately $100,000 per patient. Is this a breakthrough or a sure course for bankrupting our country? Those 500,000 people who had drug costs exceeding $50,000 in a year account for a very large percentage of the *total* cost of prescriptions in the US, certainly far out of proportion to the small part of the population they represent.

Now have I been teasing you? Offered you something and then didn't give it to you? SEX! I started this chapter talking about paying for sex and I haven't said a thing about sex since. Do I have to watch the news only to be bombarded with commercials about pills that treat penises that can't stand up? And by the way, one of those pills costs $38. That's $38 each! Another costs about $400 for a month's supply. And then I have to hear about painful sex and vaginas and the medication for women post menopause. Then I have to watch women in bed, with throaty voices and wearing sexy nightgowns telling me about erectile dysfunction. And I sure as hell hope the battery on the timer doesn't break, because after 4 hours, you can be in serious trouble.

I am also tired of old golfers telling me about blood thinners but not telling me they cost between $378 and $474 a month! Talk about *bleeding* you dry! But this blood thinner doesn't require blood tests.

Another ad is with a model who has had moderate to severe plaque psoriasis for most of her life and she tells you how few injections she needs each year to treat her psoriasis. She forgets to mention the medication costs $53,000 a year. And the ads for one of the other psoriasis medications forgot to mention that their company has the top selling drug in the world with sales of $12.54 billion in 2014. Not to mention that was a 17.7% increase in sales from 2013. Wonder if the drug reps who are trying to get to my office have played a role in that sales increase? Or the TV ads—have they increased sales?

One drug on TV is for bipolar disease. As far as I can tell, it promotes both depression *and* mania. At a cost of $950 a month ($11,400 a year) it seemingly makes the patient more depressed and the CEO of the company more manic.

And what about that *down with* lady? She might be down with something since she's always shaking her booty in the commercial. I hope she ain't down with an STD. Even if she is, the CEO of the company that makes that *down with* drug is laughing all the way to the bank. I think I just saw him driving a fleet of dump trucks to the bank. He needs a fleet of dump trucks since he sold $5.87 billion dollars worth of this *down with* drug. My calculator doesn't even have enough spaces to divide $5,870,000,000 by 10,000. That's the number of stacks of $100 bills that he needs to drive to the bank. 587,000 stacks of $100 bills! And now my calculator is broken!

Dry eyes. Wasn't there some guy with a nasal voice and dry tone who used to ask, "Do you have dry eyes?" Well, if he invested in the company making one prescription dry eye drug advertised on television, his ears just perked up since it costs $450 a month to use it. Maybe you just have to look at the price tag of the drug....the tears will start flowing if you don't have insurance and your dry eyes might not be so dry after all.

Congress passed a law that doesn't allow me to buy an incandescent light bulb (at free market value). Have they passed one that overrides the FDA's ruling in 1997 that relaxed the federal rules for direct to consumer advertising?

Drug-makers in 2014 spent $4.5 billion marketing prescription drugs, up from $3.5 billion in 2012. Obviously sex sells. If it didn't, the two most common erectile dysfunction drugs wouldn't rank in the top 5 drugs that are being advertised the most to consumers according to Kantar Media (as reported in *The Washington Post*).

Why is the United States one of the only countries (the only other one I found was New Zealand) that allows direct to consumer advertising? Clearly, such advertising encourages use of the most costly treatments, instead of less expensive treatments that would be just as effective. And how much has the pharmaceutical industry given to political campaigns? Hmmmm. How much!

To summarize, in the United States we currently have the following scenarios:

1. Medicare is not allowed to negotiate prices. They have to pay exactly what the drug companies charge for any drug.

2. In 2014, the top 25 drugs had revenues of $145 billion dollars.

3. The top selling drug pulled in $12.54 billion dollars in 2014, a 17.7% increase versus 2013.

4. $4.53 billion dollars was spent on direct to consumer advertising of drugs in 2014. A number approximately 5 times that was spent on sales forces to promote their drugs to physicians. These sales forces are now in Hawaii on two week, all-expense-paid trips.

5. The number of drugs costing over $100,000 a year tripled between 2013 and 2014.

6. 500,000+ people in the US had drug costs exceeding $50,000 in 2014.

7. It costs $1125 a day to treat hepatitis C and you have to take the drug in question for 12 weeks.

8. In 2010 the most expensive medication in the world cost $409,500 for a year's supply. This drug treats a rare condition and is termed an orphan drug. Orphan drugs can gain marketing approval more easily than most drugs and seemingly have no restriction on their price either. Perhaps they are also called orphan drugs because if you have to pay for one, you'll kill yourself and your children will be orphans.

9. The same medication sold in the United States often

costs multiples more than when it is sold in other advanced countries, such as Switzerland.

10. The rep who used to call on my office and sold the medication I use to treat pre-cancers of the skin lost his job. This was the drug that went from $110 a dose to $300 a dose in a period of about 10 years. Don't feel sorry for this rep. He cashed out about $250,000 of profit on his stock options after working for the company for 8 years. He took 6 months off to play and figure out the next company he should work for.

11. If you don't have insurance, you ain't gettin any (sex) if the pill you need costs $38.

And what about the reps who try to call on my office? They are part of a yearly expenditure of $24 billion dollars by the pharmaceutical industry (2012). Added to the direct to consumer marketing dollars, it seems pretty likely that more is spent on marketing than on research and development.

A 2013 report by FiercePharma collected data from Nielsen and estimated that 80 drug ads air every hour of every day on American television. It seems that half of those 80 are on during the 6:30 p.m. news every night in my location. The other half are on any other time I am watching television.

Now I'd hate to end this chapter without at least getting one legal jab in. So one night I was watching TV and they were talking about testosterone replacement drugs. As if erectile dysfunction drugs and painful vagina drugs aren't enough, I have to hear about testosterone problems too. So the ad was the usual one about have you or a family member been harmed or killed by a testosterone replacement drug? You know how these ads go. Call 1-800-BAD DRUG. I was in a good mood. Time to call.

I got the phone, dialed, and when they answered, I said, "Is this 1-800-BAD-LAWYER?"

Seemingly seriously they replied, "No, it's 1-800-BAD DRUG."

I told them, "Sorry, I got the wrong number."

I called back and said, "I just saw the TV commercial and my favorite uncle died from testosterone replacement."

"Oh, we are *soooooo* sorry to har that."

I asked if they wanted to hear the story (I knew they were salivating on the other end so I kept it serious and entertaining at the same time).

"Well, my uncle, you know, he couldn't perform. So he went to the doctor and he had his testosterone checked and sure enough it was low. So they put him on one of those testosterone drugs you rub on your skin. Sure enough, in no time he was ready to go. Well, he hired himself this prostitute. And boy, she was *reaaaallll* good looking. They got to the hotel and she took her clothes off and he was *reaaaallll* ready, if you know what I mean. Well, he had the best sex of his life, and right after, he had a massive heart attack and died."

"Oh, we are so sorry to hear that. How old was your uncle?"

I told them that he was 80.

"Sorry, we only take cases of people 60 or under."

Then they hung up on me.

And the red box of chocolates I got so I could forget about the Black Box warning of the drug?

They didn't even taste that good!

Chapter 27

Farting in The Amazon

The opportunity to travel to 37 countries has allowed me to see a multitude of visually stunning things. While the world's natural beauty has etched amazing images in my mind, two of these images stand out more than any others. Those two are of people whom I observed.

The first image is a woman paddling a canoe in the Peruvian Amazon within a region known as the Pacaya Samaria Reserve. She was smiling. Unbeknownst to her, I took her photo. Later, when I looked at the photo, I thought about her smile. I know she did not see me taking her photo. I was far away from her and I was not in her line of vision. I have no idea where she came from or where she was going.

Perhaps she was going to a nearby village to pick up food for her family? I thought to myself, why was she smiling? Had I farted, and she was laughing because I farted? No, I hadn't farted. Did I crack a great joke and she was laughing? No, I hadn't even cracked a bad joke. Remember, she hadn't seen me and we never communicated with one another. She was just smiling.

This smile made me think of something simple, yet profound. What do you need to be happy? Remember the first chapter where I wrote about life being simpler in the 1970s and 1980s, the time period before the advent of the internet, email, cell phones, texting, and the like? Most parts of the Amazon still vastly predate the development of the United States in the 1970s and 1980s. The majority of people living along the Amazon River live in villages. Their homes are huts. They farm basic foods, hunt, and fish and they trade for things they need. In the end, they have shelter, food, and companionship.

Do you really need more than that? Certainly this woman in the canoe likely lived her life with little, undeniably much less than what I have. The absence of those things that likely complicate my life (and yours if you are reading this) did not detract whatsoever from the happiness I observed in her. I recall the peace and the vastness of the Amazon. I also recall the absence of the internet, cell phones, and virtually any capacity to connect to the world while I was there. It was the only time in a decade and a half that I was fully disconnected. The lack of technology produced a profound peace within me. Seemingly, her lack of it produced the same feeling in her. Less really is more.

The second image is that of a man begging on a crowded street in Vienna, Austria. He was sitting on the street, his back up against a stainless steel public garbage can with a cup in his hand. He was not smiling, yet he did not look unhappy either. He seemed calm and perhaps even content. Like the woman paddling her canoe in the Amazon, he did not know that I took his photo. I was rather far away from him when I took it.

His image made me think of sameness. That he and I are the same. We both have the same essential needs—food, shelter, and companionship. I also saw the sameness in that I could be in the same position that he was in or he could be in mine with a few changes of circumstances. I felt truly equal to him, despite my greater resources. I wondered who he really was and why he was begging? Perhaps he was once a famous professor at the University of Vienna? Maybe he got laid off? Divorced? Became ill? Bankrupt? Maybe something happened to him that could happen to me? Again, I saw equality, the feeling that the two of us were really the same. It reminded me that both of us were human beings and that no human being is better or superior to any other.

When I returned home and looked at his photo again, something even more profound hit me. While he was in need (begging) I hadn't given him anything, yet while I had pretty much everything I needed, he had given something amazing to ME, namely, this understanding of our sameness and equality. My impact to him, a big fat zero. But his impact to me, immeasurable. I've shown his photo at talks I've given to the community, to youth groups, and I've also shared it with many patients. I've told this story over and over. He'll probably never know the positive impact he has had on the world.

Another lesson—never forget the *unintended* impact you have on other people's lives.

For photos of the woman in the canoe and the man in Vienna check

www.149waystowipeyourass.com/images

Standing "O"

To Buster: A Man of great character. I want you to teach me how to ride a Harley when I get to heaven.

To Neil: Once a great friend, always a great friend.

To Dan (the plumber): Shame on you!

To an old man at the VA hospital: You called me out. I **AM** a Wisenheimer.

To Johnson, the boat repair guy: Thanks for nothing. I mean thanks for giving me a good title for a chapter in my book.

To STRIKEOUT: If I ever become a pitcher, I suggest you don't go to bat.

To SMOOT: I hope you had a long and wonderful life after that episode at the West Los Angeles VA Hospital in 1992.

To Dr. Mitchell: For sustained friendship, memories, and laughs for more than 20 years.

To WEINER: Thanks for having a great last name.

To TJ: Thanks for teaching me something valuable and standing up for what is right.

To Fred: I promise to try my hardest to make you smile every time I see you.

To Mr. Whalley: You brought calm to me while you were alive and every day after your passing. Thank you for serving our country in WWII.

To Chan: If you drive to my house, I've got a $20 tip for you.

To Mr. Kraft: I hope I was able to provide you a small amount of comfort during your valiant fight.

To Dr. Gerding: Thank you for providing me the absolute certainty that medicine was my calling.

To Bruno: Thank you for knowing when to take the training wheels off.

To CWRU: Thanks for providing me a great education and allowing me to get it without taking on any debt.

To Dan Batzel: Thank you for repeatedly encouraging me to consider California for my medical education and sharing numerous "Polish Boys" with me.

To US Airways: First, before telling you thank you, this might be the only time anyone has ever thanked an airline for anything—Thank you for giving me the free ticket that changed my life. In an almost past-life experience I flew on US Airways' very last day of operation (October 16, 2015) to visit my parents.

To Ted: Thank you for being a big brother and uncle, being focused, and suggesting that I become a dermatologist.

To Dr. Maibach: Thank you for sharing your love and passion for dermatology.

To the psychiatry attending physicians at UCSF: Thank you for proving to me that there was no way I could ever be a psychiatrist.

To Dr. Marcus Conant: Thank you for touching my life

and 25 years later knowing that working with you was the grandest educational opportunity of my life.

To Hugh Sless and Vasteov Paper: Maybe one day you'll publish a book that actually teaches I/T to make my life easier instead of harder.

To Helga and Olga: Keep up the good work. Also, remember to bring me earplugs so I don't have to listen to any whining or crying during the next scrotal surgery.

To My Patients: Thank you for providing me so much material (often humor) to write about. Thank you also for your love and appreciation and for your life lessons shared with me. Thank you for letting me be a part of your lives and for teaching me so much. And, to a recent patient, Joey, for just being you and making me want to help you any possible way I could. Thank you for serving in Vietnam. I hope you enjoyed the Reuben sandwich and cold Budweiser.

To The Pharmaceutical Industry: Get out of my office! Get out of my conferences! And get off of my TV!

To The Woman in the Canoe and the Man in Vienna: Thank you for the impact that you never even knew you had.

To My Wife: Thank you for your love all of these years and for your tolerance, patience, kindness, beauty, sexiness, forgiveness, and example you show to me and the world and for you putting up with my amazing, uncanny, phenomenal humor—even the type that isn't funny but I can still make you laugh with it.

To Oliver (All over my heart): Thank you for being rambunctious, happy, astoundingly smart, and mostly a good boy all 3.6 pounds (one pound of ears) of amazing Papillon puppy. Oliver now weighs 8.1 pounds.

To My Parents: For bringing me into this world and providing for me. It's taken the better part of 50 years to fully understand how much you sacrificed, how hard you worked, and how great a job you did. I love you more than words can describe.

And very special thanks to three more people without whom I could not possibly have done this book:

To Carl Graves: Like Buster Williams I knew you were *the* person for the job. Your genius, flair, aptitude, imagination, acumen, ingenuity, talent, and creativity in designing the cover of this book were all spot-on (not the toilet paper)! You took an image, a concept and a brainchild and turned it into life.

To Karen Woolley-Stewart: To you I owe a level of gratitude that cannot be expressed. You took what looked like a very long term paper and beautifully, elegantly, skillfully, fastidiously, and precisely converted it into a book saving me from hysteria and insanity. You are the *queen of formatters*. I would not have a book were it not for you.

To June Robb: For proofreading my manuscript, preventing me from doing something that could have hurt myself. Likewise, for catching the 100 mistakes that I had missed.

About the Author

Steven F. Wolfe, MD was born and raised in New York City. He is a dermatologist and lives with his wife Sheri (who has somehow been able to survive his style of humor for the past 25 years) and his Papillon puppy, Oliver, (All Over My Heart) who bit his toes numerous times while he was writing *149 Ways to Wipe Your Ass*.

See the doc and his puppy at
www.149waystowipeyourass.com/bio

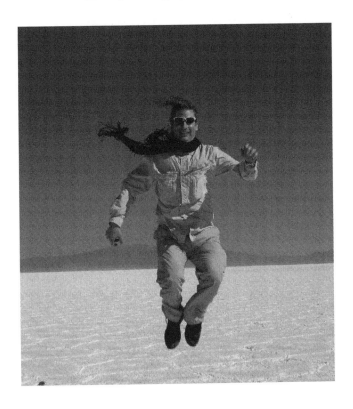

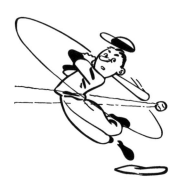

Made in the USA
Middletown, DE
30 November 2020